Childhood
Illnesses
Handbook

Childhood Illnesses Handbook

Dr Peter Rowan

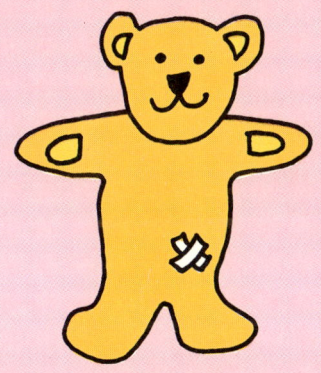

WINDWARD

For Edward and Sarah

Windward
an imprint owned by W H Smith and Son Limited
Registered no 237811 England
Trading as W H Smith Distributors
St John's House, East Street, Leicester LE1 6NE

This book was designed and produced by
Amanuensis Books Limited
12 Station Road
Didcot
Oxfordshire OX11 7LN

Editorial and art director: Loraine Fergusson
Senior editor: Lynne Gregory
Illustration: David Gifford, Coral Mula, Sue Lines, Sharon
Perks, Shona Grant
Charts: Mick Brennan, Simon Roulstone
Indexer: Susan Ramsey

Printed and bound in Portugal by Printer Portuguesa Lda

CONTENTS

Introduction

One night Sarah, my little girl, was ill with earache and she climbed into bed with us for comfort. When things were better again she thanked me and asked what happened to sick children who didn't have a doctor to climb into bed with.

This book aims to help in just this sort of situation when a child goes down with one of the common ailments which needs lots of home nursing and tender loving care. My two children are at present working their way through many of them and I have tried to write a book which I would find helpful if I was not a family doctor.

You won't find many of the rare illnesses or accidents here. It is about everyday medical problems that all parents with children face. It is not a substitute for your own family doctor, nor for the important instinct that parents have about their own children's well being. However, I hope it helps to bridge that gap between the two.

I also hope it helps when someone wakes up next to you and says "My ear hurts!"

Peter Ronan.

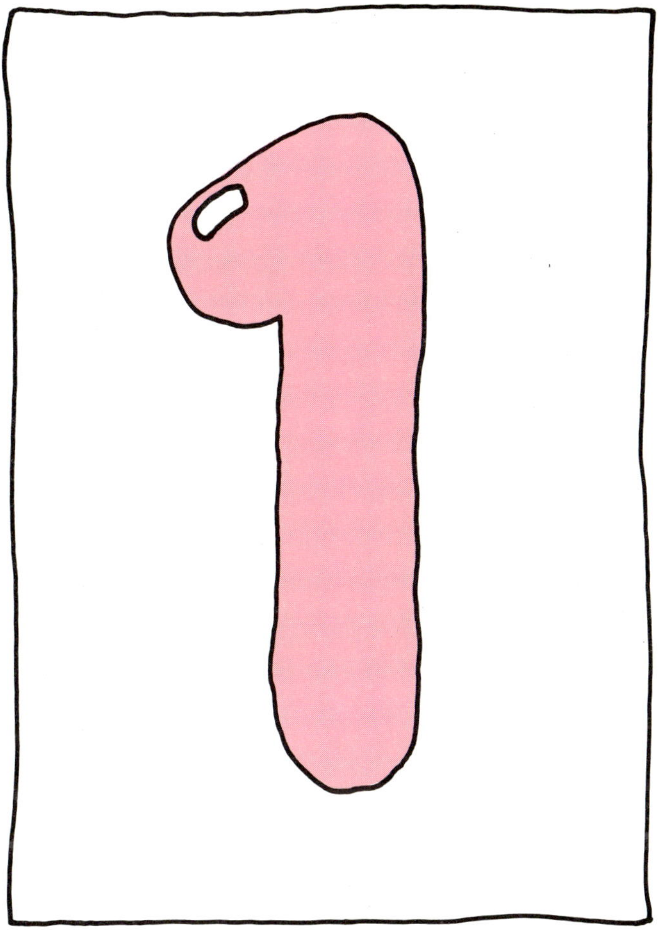

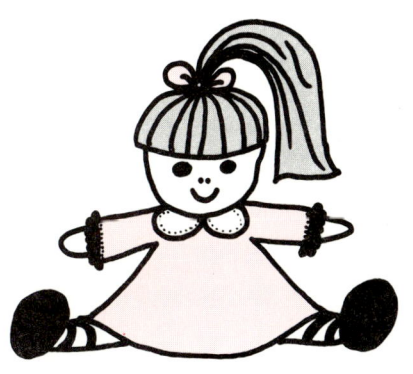

Home nursing

Right up until the end of World War II, the parents' first concern when a child fell ill was whether the child was going to live or not. Children still contract a great many illnesses, but better nutrition, general health and drugs such as antibiotics mean that these diseases are no longer life-threatening in the Western world. Most can be nursed at home, and even though parents know the child will make a full recovery, it does not make the task of home nursing any less stressful. Children are not easy patients.

Bedrest

Take your doctor's advice about this but keep the child comfortable somewhere where you can keep an eye and ear open. Sick children need plenty of attention. Bedrooms tend to be rather isolated parts of the house out of the mainstream of family life. It is rarely necessary to confine a child to bed and in my experience children are much happier wrapped up in a makeshift bed on the sofa in front of the television. The room is warm and the child can enjoy the hub-bub of life going on around him or her.

Warmth or fresh air

If the child has a temperature it needs to be brought down, not stoked up. Overheating can cause febrile convulsions (see page 38). When a child has a temperature make sure the room is warm but that the child is not prevented from losing heat by wearing too many warm clothes.

Eating and drinking

A child who is ill for a few days with one of the common childhood illnesses is likely to go off food, especially if the illness is associated with feeling sick anyway. Do not worry about this temporary loss of appetite.

Drinking is another matter altogether. The child must be encouraged to drink more than enough to replace any fluid that is being lost as sweat or as diarrhoea. (See chart page 102-3). Vary drinks to make them interesting and give the child small amounts to drink as often as possible. This is especially effective if the child feels sick. The actual drink itself is not critical but fresh fruit drinks are popular with children and are nutritionally well-balanced. Let the child choose. Special mixtures are available for diarrhoea and vomiting (see page 101).

Very young children usually take their fluids from a teacher beaker. If not they too should regularly be given small amounts by spoon.

Once the child starts to feel hungry again start him or her off with small amounts of a favourite food. Ice creams, jellies and cool yoghurt (let the child order the flavour if possible) are very good if there is a sore throat. Avoid milky foods, however, if there has been a tummy upset because this may cause diarrhoea again.

Giving medicine

There is an element of truth in the belief that the more effective a medicine the worse it tastes. Paracetamol is a good example. For this reason children's medicine is prepared with flavouring to encourage the child to take it. Sometimes, however, the added flavours or the texture of the elixir do not appeal to a child or the medicine itself is simply too difficult to disguise.

Other ways of getting the child to take the medicine then have to be found. If they come in tablet form crush the tablets and mix with jam or something similar and feed this to the child on a spoon or wash down with some fruit juice. The taste of liquid medicine can be made more appealing by mixing it with a diluted fruit juice. In the end, however,

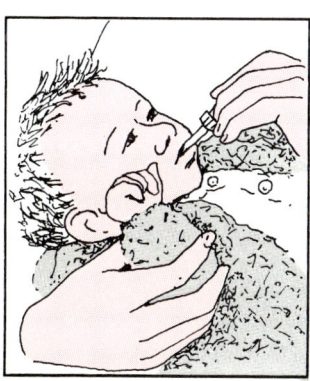

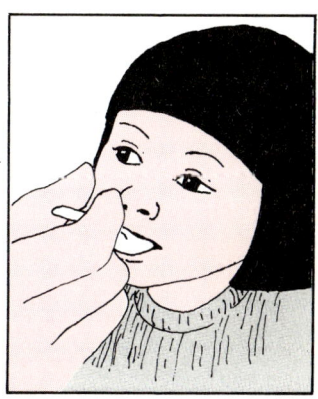

Use a dropper to give medicine to a small baby. Modern preparations are usually very sweet and most babies take them readily.

Before giving medicine, assume your child is going to enjoy it. Often the medicine tastes so good that the problem is ignoring the demands for more.

you may have to resort to a blend of firmness and bribery (the promise of something nice afterwards) which will require all your persuasive powers.

It is sometimes necessary to hold a young child down to get a spoonful of medicine in and an extra pair of hands could well come in useful. Be both firm and gentle. A wriggling baby is fairly easily held still by being wrapped in a blanket. Hold the child's head up so that there is no danger of the medicine making the child choke.

Use spoons and droppers to get the medicine into the mouth or measure out the dose into an egg cup, dip your finger in and allow the baby to suck the medicine off it. This takes time but will often work when other ways are not being well received.

Do not worry about the mess caused by medicine missing the mouth or being dribbled out. Just ensure that the correct dose is actually given in the end. Sticky medicines have the advantage of being more difficult than watery liquids to spit out!

Points to remember

● Always give medicines as advised by the doctor and make sure important courses of medicines are finished.
● If the doctor gives you more than the medicine make sure you know which ones must be finished and which can be stopped when the child is better.
● Check the label and dose just before giving.
● Keep a clear record of doses given and tape it up somewhere near where you store the medicine. It is not easy to give a week's course of an antibiotic with doses up to three or four times a day without a reminder and checklist.
● Put the top back securely on the bottle of medicine and put it away out of reach.
● Do not store half-used courses of drugs like antibiotics for use the next time. Empty them down the lavatory before throwing the bottles away.
● Make sure medicines, like asthma inhalers, which are used intermittently are kept up to date and that you have an extra supply in case medicines are lost or you run out at weekends.
● It is useful to have double supplies of things like inhalers: one to be kept at home, the other at school.

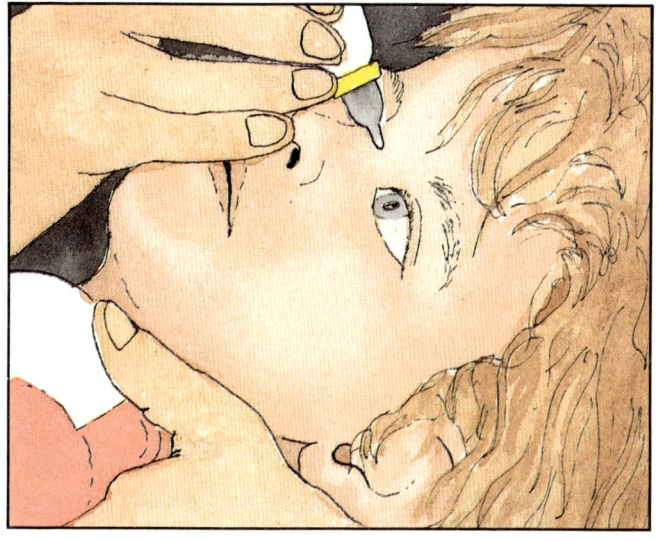

When giving a child eye drops, make sure that the head is tipped to one side so that fluid from the treated eye does not run across the face into the other eye.

Giving eye medicines

Apply the cream or drops to the area between the lower lid and the eye itself. Young babies should be held. Keep the child's head tilted to the same side as the eye being treated so that fluid does not run into the other eye which can spread the infection. Similarly, the dropper or tube should not come into contact with the eye.

Eye medicines do not usually sting when they are applied and are often most useful at night. Your doctor will decide if a particular drug is given in drop or ointment form. Ointments are rather sticky but have the advantage that they do not run out of the eye.

As with other medicines throw eye medicines away once they have been opened and used and do not treat another child who appears to go down with the same problem with the same medicine.

Isolation

This is rarely necessary nowadays. Most infectious diseases are passed on before they are diagnosed and there is little point in protecting a child from these almost inevitable diseases of childhood. Many childhood diseases are much more serious in adulthood, for example mumps. Now that children are being vaccinated against German measles and mumps, isolation has become even less important.

There are important exceptions to this. Meningitis and hepatitis are conditions which do need isolation and these children will probably be looked after in hospital. Children with German measles should be kept away from pregnant mothers unless the mother's blood test for immunity (usually checked in early pregnancy) is known to be positive. Take your doctor's advice if you have any worries about the infectiousness of your child.

Games

Children with one of the common childhood illnesses are rarely ill for more than a few days. Once they start to get better they will want to be amused and to play.

The games and toys that are often the most comfort are the ones which have been put aside as the child has grown up and out of them. Not only is there an element of novelty about an old toy or a forgotten game, but the child finds it comforting to go back a few months in time to play with something tried and trusted.

In an ideal world the parent would have the patience of a saint and masses of time to devote to caring for the child. In reality this is unlikely so spend time with the child but make it short and enthusiastic. This is far better than begrudging an hour when the child knows you are not enjoying their company. I find television a great help during the child's convalescence. A new or favourite old video is one of the best and most appreciated of treats you can give a sick child. Especially so if you let the child watch it at times which are normally out of hours. Not every parent is enthusiastic about television and videos (some do not even have them) and this is obviously a matter of individual choice.

When I was ill as a child my parents used to let me look through the family encylopaedia without its dull brown cover on. This extraordinary treat made a tremendous difference to the books and kept me interested for hours as a result. Try to find something new and special like this for the child, perhaps something of yours that they are not normally allowed to play with.

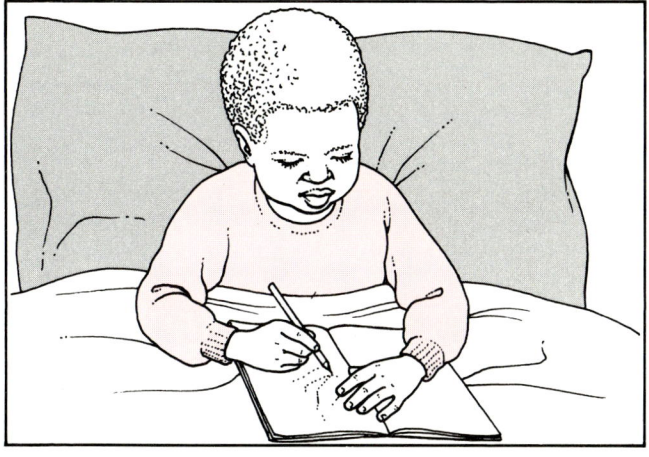

Invest in a new drawing book and set of pencils because the novelty may be enough to keep a bedridden child content.

Family medicine chest

It is a very good idea for a family to have a basic box which contains everything that would be needed in an emergency. If all medicines, lotions, creams and bandages are kept together it should make them easier to locate and to keep up-to-date. Keep the box out of the reach of children and in a warm room. (Medicines store better at a constant temperature.) A top cupboard in the kitchen is often a good first choice in most houses.

The list below is a rough guide to the possible contents of a family medicine chest. It is impossible to include medicines for every eventuality, after all your house is not a hospital, but if you do find that something useful is missing on one occasion make a note and ensure it is there for next time.

Preparations
1. Paracctamol clixir for children under six, soluble paracetamol tablets for older children
2. Sachets of rehydrating mixtures ready to make up
3. Prescribed medicines that are not carried by the child (e.g. asthma preparations)
4. An antiseptic cream
5. Calamine lotion
6. Antihistamine cream for stings

Warm Climates
eg Northern Europe

First three days	SPF 10 Water resistant
Next three days	SPF 8 Water resistant
Subsequent days	SPF 6 Water resistant

A tan is the skin's natural protection against harmful ultraviolet rays, but it must be allowed to develop gradually. If the skin goes red or peels, then damage has occurred. If your child's skin can

Items
1. Two sizes of crepe bandaging (10cm and 5cm) and a selection of cotton bandages
2. Adhesive tape
3. Selection of waterproof plasters
4. Scissors and tweezers
5. Cotton wool
6. Safety pins
7. Two mercury thermometers and a strip thermometer for the forehead
8. A 5ml plastic spoon

These boxes can be made up or bought. Stick emergency numbers, such as your doctor's and that of the local hospital, inside the lid. If you are not on the phone ensure you have some loose change in the box for the pay phone.

Hot Climates

eg Mediterranean,
Canaries, Africa

First three days

SPF 12
Water resistant

SPF 15 on shoulders lips
backs of neck etc

Next three days

SPF 10
Water resistant

Subsequent days

SPF 10
Water resistant

withstand ten minutes of sun without redenning, he or she can withstand two and a half hours when protected with SPF 15 (10 minutes x 15).

Holiday medicines

The following list is a guide to what you might consider taking on holiday.

1. Rehydrating mixtures in case of diarrhoea and vomiting
2. Paracetamol elixir
3. Travel sickness medicines (see below)
4. Sun screen in appropriate strengths for your children and your destination
5. Other items from your medicine cabinet which you know from experience you may need e.g. calamine

Babies on holiday

Do not be afraid to take very young babies on holiday. You are the best judge as to whether a holiday abroad will suit your children. In general though there is no reason why they should be protected from exotic holidays abroad.

My own son took his first holiday in the Indian Ocean at the age of three months. He slept contentedly in his sky cot for most of the 13-hour flight and once there was the one least bothered by the change in food and water as he was being breast fed. Gastroenteritis is more of a risk in bottle fed children so be extra vigilant in cleaning and sterilizing the baby's feeding equipment and store in clean plastic bags. Most problems such as sunburn, tummy upsets and travel sickness can be avoided or easily dealt with.

Travel sickness
Not all children who are sick in cars, boats and planes are in fact motion sick. It is a common problem, however, which is unusual before six months and at its peak amongst ten year olds. Most children grow out of the problem but there are ways in which the trouble can be reduced.

Keep the child occupied when travelling. Play games which make the child look out of the window because with a view of the horizon the brain seems to cope better with the messages it is receiving about the body's changing position and this reduces the possibility of motion sickness.

There are medicines available which also help. Consult your doctor or pharmacist to ensure that you get the best medicine for the particular journey your child is going to make. A cross-channel ferry journey will require a different medicine to an air flight to Australia. The most effective travel sickness medicines contain an antihistamine which may make the child drowsy which is an added benefit.

There are some sensible rules which apply when giving your child travel sickness medicine.

● Do not let your child have a large or spicy meal just before travelling. Make sure, however, that there is a light snack available for the child to eat on the journey as it may actually help.
● Give the child the medicine before he or she starts to feel sick. Some preparations should be given a few hours before the start of the journey.
● Play the problem down. If the child does not think about being sick then very often the nausea will not begin. Any non-medical remedies which seem to work with the child are also well worth pursuing even if they seem completely illogical (such as sitting the child on a brown paper bag).

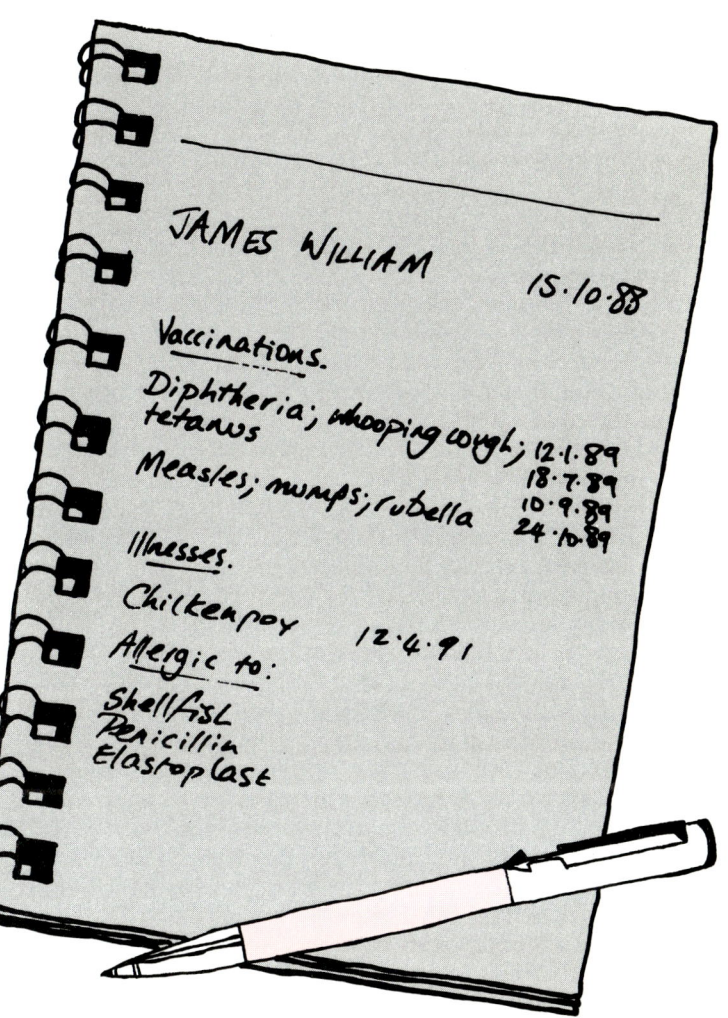

JAMES WILLIAM   15·10·88

Vaccinations.

Diphtheria; whooping cough; 12·1·89
tetanus   18·7·89
Measles; mumps; rubella   10·9·89
                      24·10·89

Illnesses.

Chickenpox   12·4·91

Allergic to:

Shellfish
Penicillin
Elastoplast

Keeping a record

Details about the childhood illnesses can get forgotten over time. Confusion over the type of disease and even which child was affected does arise so it is well worth keeping a medical record of each serious illness.

When a child starts a new school, this information is often asked for.

Visiting the doctor

Consult your family doctor if you are at all worried about your child's health. It is difficult for a book to be precise about what is and what is not an emergency or indeed when a child requires a home visit. There are, however, some useful general guidelines.

Emergency calls

At some time you will have to call a doctor who is not familiar with your family out of hours. It helps a great deal if you can calmly explain what is wrong. Remember the doctor may not know details which you take for granted like the child's age, for example. Be prepared to give the following information about the sick child early on in your request for advice or a visit:

● The child's age and sex
● The main reasons for your concern. This may seem an obvious thing to say but a parent is often too wrapped up in the child's problem to be short and concise. The doctor will ask for details once the problem is outlined.
● The timing of events e.g. "My four-year-old girl is normally well but for three days she has been off food and an hour ago she complained of a bellyache which is getting worse."
● The treatment, if any, that the child has received so far including details about prescribed medicines.
● Your address with directions. Remember some homes can be difficult for a doctor to find if unfamiliar with the area, especially at night. Relate your directions to local landmarks like pubs and churches. An outside light in the dead of night can be like a beacon. Leave a phone number at which you can be contacted. If you have rung the doctor from a call box, give your pay phone number immediately so that if you run out of coins you can be rung back.

Home visits

Ask for a home visit if you think the child is too ill to make the journey to the surgery or you have no means of getting there. Consider whether the child is infectious and should be kept away from other sick people. Ask for advice from the surgery by phone. It helps the doctor to organize the day's work if non-urgent visits are requested before about mid-morning.

A temperature is not a sufficient reason not to take the child out to the surgery if he or she can be wrapped up warmly and taken by car. After all, if your child was seriously ill you would not hesitate taking him or her to hospital if your doctor advised it.

Helping the doctor
A good working relationship between you and your doctor will help enormously. When visiting the surgery be prepared to give him or her a clear story of what you have noticed is wrong with the child and what is worrying you. Be prepared to answer questions that may not at first seem relevant. You may find it helpful to have a written list of points relating to the child's illness so that no detail is forgotten. The doctor may wish to know details dating back several days and it can be very difficult to remember them accurately.

Dress the child in loose clothing which is easy to remove for thorough investigation of chests and tummies, front and back. If you baby is in disposable nappies, bring a spare — the doctor may need to take the existing one off.

Specialists
The practice of medicine is not an exact science and opinion probably differs at general practice level more than any other. This does not mean that one opinion is wrong and another right, just that different doctors approach problems in different ways. A good doctor never minds referring you to a colleague or specialist if you need the reassurance of another opinion.

Going to hospital

This can be a frightening experience for a child despite the fact that nowadays children's wards are much friendlier places than they used to be. Here are some tips to help make the child's stay as trouble-free as possible.

● There are many children's books available illustrating what a child can expect when he or she goes into hospital. Buy one or borrow one from your local library if you can. Read it with your child like any other bedtime story.
● Talk honestly to the child before he or she goes in. Try and explain simply what is happening and why. Reassure the child that things will be better for the visit and put the emphasis on the homecoming.

● If your child is under the age of about six you should be able to arrange to stay in hospital as well. Ask the sister or staff nurse on the children's ward beforehand. They should also be able to answer any questions you have before the child is admitted.

● Gather together some favourite old toys for the child to play with. Play is important therapy for children in hospital just as at home. Familiar objects in an unfamiliar place are very reassuring.

● Make sure someone close to the child is available to be with him or her for most of the stay.

● When the child comes out of hospital be firm about getting back into a normal routine. It usually takes a little time to readjust to home life and the child may actually miss the excitement, company and toys of the hospital ward.

● Take with you all the medicines your child is using both regularly and from time to time.

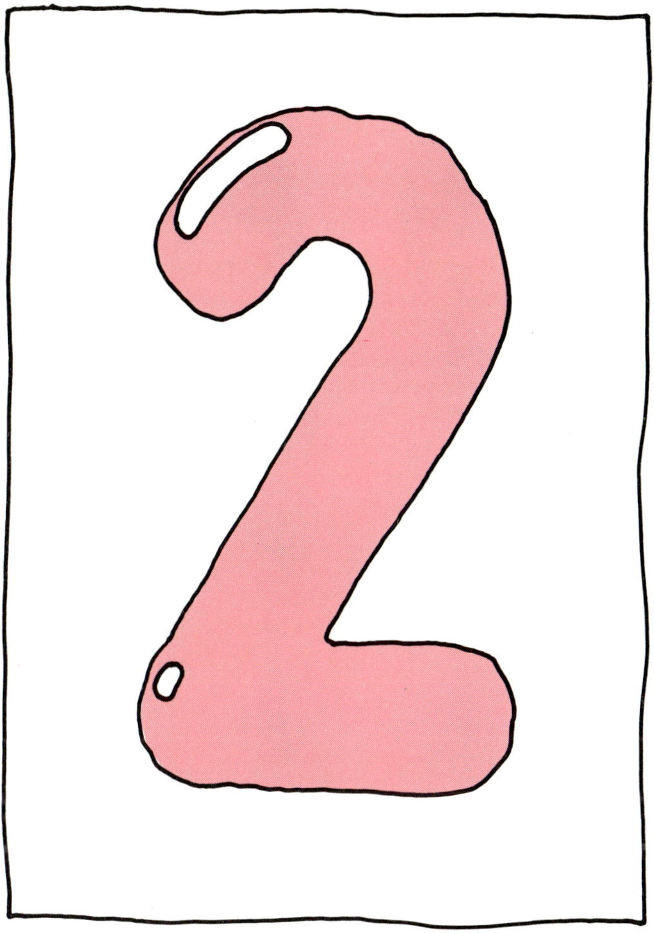

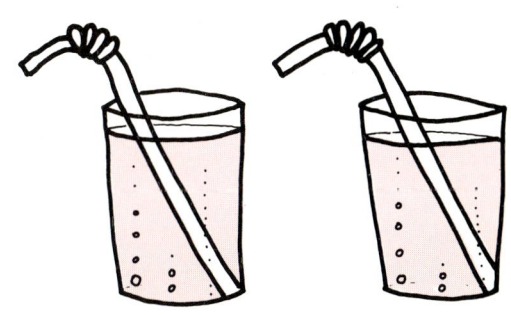

Childhood diseases

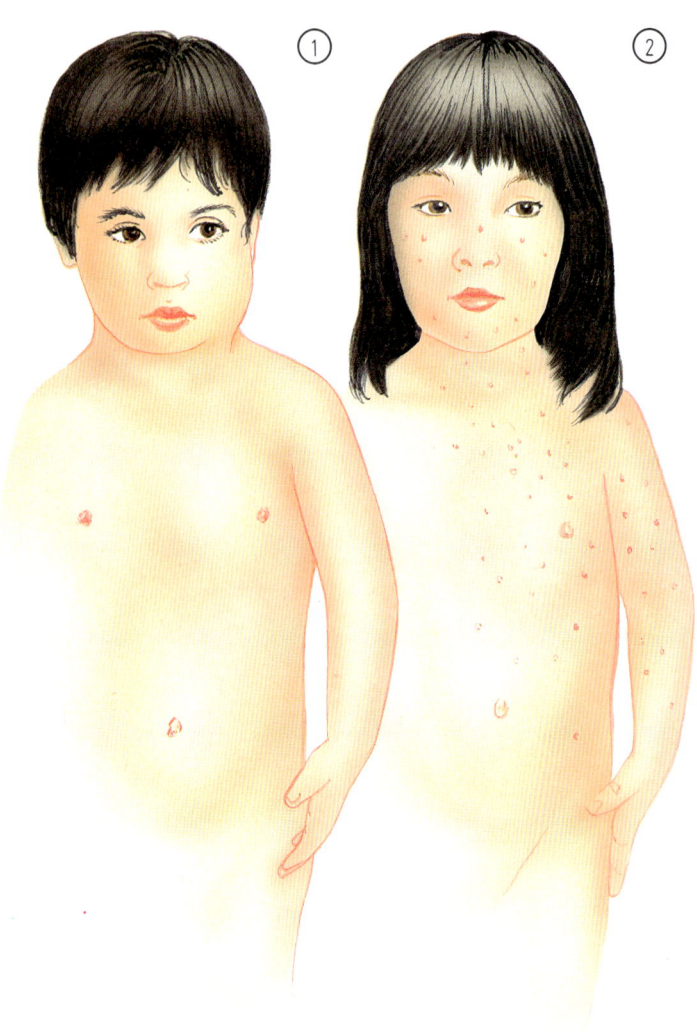

1. **Mumps** p 27-29
   see also p 34-5, 82,
   156-7
2. **Chickenpox** p 24-5
   see also p 34-5, 156-7
3. **German measles** p 25-6
   see also p 12, 34-5,
   156-7
   Roseola infantum p 33

4. **Measles** p 29-30
   see also p 23, 51, 34-5,
   156-7

Whopping cough p 31-3
see also 34-5, 51, 156-7
Meningitis p 36-7
see also p 12, 40
Febrile convulsion p 38-9

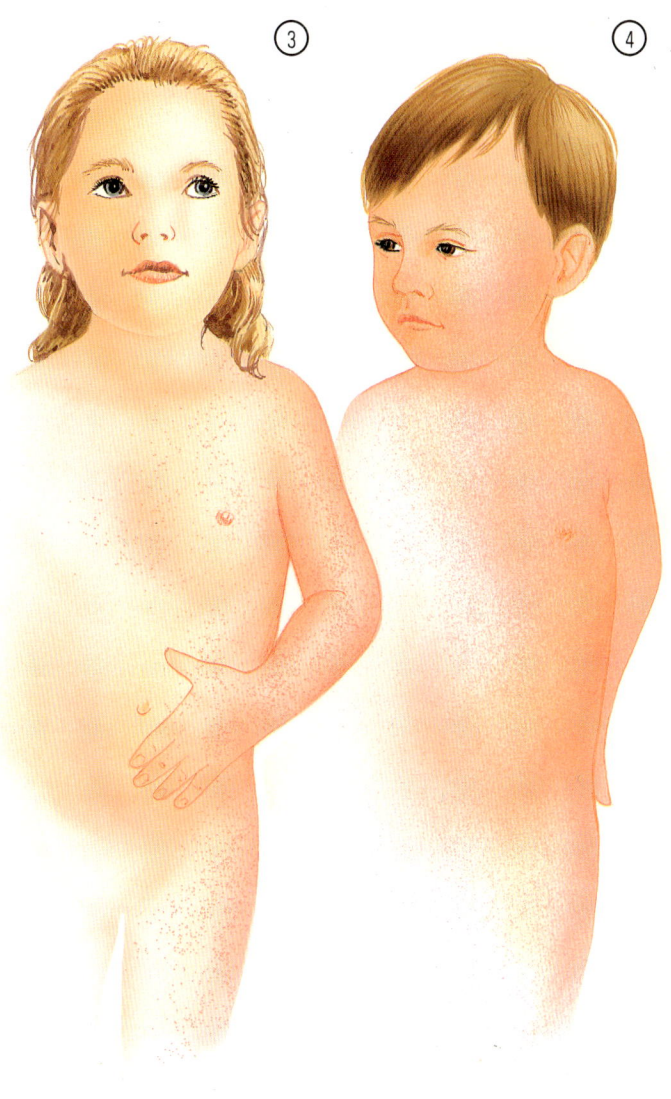

Childhood diseases

There are some diseases which are so infectious that they are usually caught when we are young. Sometimes a child is ill with one and it may be difficult even to give it a name. Many, but not all, are caused by viruses which can spread like wildfire through a family, a class at school, or a whole community of people. With others, only one member of the family will get it.

Some of these diseases can be prevented by vaccination. As a general rule, once you have had your bout of a particular illness, you will not get it again because your body has built up an immunity to that germ, although this varies from child to child and with each particular illness.

Chickenpox

In children, chickenpox is one of the mildest childhood diseases but also one which is most easily caught, therefore it usually affects children under the age of ten.

Cause
It is caused by a virus identical to the one that causes shingles. It spreads by airborn droplets as well as from the spots on the skin. Patients with shingles can give someone chickenpox, but it does not work the other way around. A child with chickenpox cannot give a grandparent shingles.

Signs and symptoms
The illness usually begins with a fever and very soon after this comes the itchy rash. The spots are small and raised but develop into inflamed, fluid-filled blisters which finally crust over. They appear in crops, so in the middle of the illness there will be spots at different stages of development, some just appearing, others crusting over, the earliest ones healing up. The rash is a central one, the spots tending to be on the trunk of the body. However,

During a bout of German measles the lymph glands behind the ear enlarge.

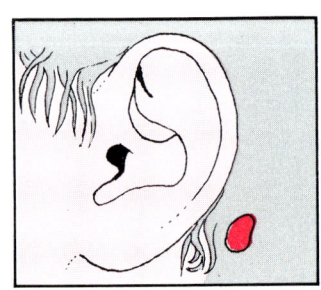

they often spread to the face, arms and legs. They should heal without scars.

Complications
These are not common in healthy children. The commonest problem is that the itchy spots get their tops scratched off allowing bacteria from the skin to enter and cause infection. It also makes scars more of a possibility.

Treatment
Chickenpox is usually a fairly mild illness. The main problems come from the skin, so careful attention to the spots is important. Relieve the itching with frequent coats of calamine and when bathing your child, add an antiseptic to the water. It makes sense to keep the child's finger nails as short as possible and to try and see mittens are worn at night. If the child resists, wait until he or she is asleep and then put the gloves on. Spots in the mouth can be relieved by a mouth wash.

If things get bad, the itching can be treated by one of the antihistamine syrups such as promethazine (Phenergan) or trimeprazine (Vallergan). These have the added advantage of making the child feel more sleepy if given before bedtime, as well as relieving the itching. Rarely children may develop chickenpox spots in their lungs which makes them cough, but this is more common in adults.

Prevention
There is rarely a need to give healthy children any protection from chickenpox. Once you have had it, you are immune for life.

German measles

German measles is usually a very mild illness these days, and is caused by the rubella virus which is spread through the air in infected droplets of moisture. It is unimportant in children, but devastating in pregnant women.

Signs and symptoms
The illness usually starts with a slight fever, rash and enlarged glands. One of the characteristics of rubella is that some lymph glands behind the ear and towards the back of the neck below the hairline can enlarge. These can be felt as hard little lumps beneath the scalp. The child may also have a sore throat and inflamed eyes.

The flat, light pink rash starts on the face and neck and quickly spreads to the trunk. It comes out about 24 hours after the child starts to feel ill and lasts between six hours to a couple of days.

Having looked at a classic case of rubella, it has to be said that many cases are so mild that they pass simply as another childhood viral illness. The rash, for example, may go unnoticed. For this reason your family doctor may be unwilling to state definitely that a child has had German measles. This is a wise move because later in life it is very important for a girl to know if she is immune to the virus.

Complications
It is ironic that a mild childhood illness (much less unpleasant than say measles) can have such dreadful effects on an unborn baby. If a woman in the first four months of the pregnancy catches German measles the baby runs the risk of being born with defects to many parts of the body including the heart, the eyes in the form of cataracts and the ears in the form of deafness. Sometimes the deformities are so severe that the baby miscarries or dies soon after being born. Nowadays the situation is preventable, so this tragedy should never happen.

A woman who is immune to rubella, either because she caught it as a child, or because she has been vaccinated against it, will not get German measles and her unborn baby is therefore safe. Unfortunately, at present about one in five girls reaching childbearing age are liable to go down with this virus. Low immunity can be identified with a blood test and protection given, but the problem is that many women are still at risk before they get pregnant. Parents must make sure that their girls reach puberty without slipping through the net.

As I've said, it is not easy to diagnose German measles without blood tests and it is not enough simply to have seen a rash years ago during a mild viral illness. It is not surprising that many doctors will not commit themselves to a definite diagnosis when a little girl over the age of five who has not had the benefit of the new pre-school vaccination program has possible German measles.

If a child is suspected of having German measles, he or she should be kept away from women in the early stage of pregnancy unless they know they are immune. All women are tested in early pregnancy but newly pregnant women should check their status by asking their doctor.

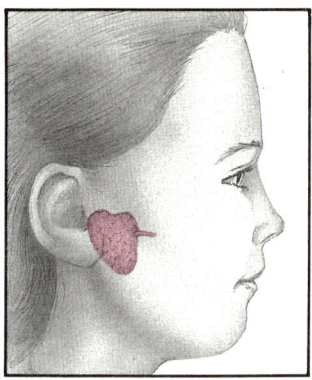

The parotid gland lies over the lower jaw bone just below the ear. The mumps virus causes this gland to swell producing the characteristic swelling of the face.

Mumps

Mumps is caused by a virus which spreads from person to person through small contaminated water droplets in the air. It affects children mainly between the ages of five and fifteen. In fact it is not common in the under fives. Because it is less infectious than some of the other diseases such as measles and chickenpox, there is more chance of missing it as a child. It is not uncommon to get mumps in adulthood when it can be a more severe illness.

Signs and symptoms
The virus affects various parts of the body but the most vunerable appears to be the parotid salivary glands which lie under the skin on each side of the face at the angle of the jaw. Many people (25%)have mumps without knowing it; but usually a child feels ill for a few days before one or both of these glands start to swell making your poor child look like a miserable doormouse. The natural hollow behind the lower jaw is filled in. This swelling is usually the main sign in a case of mumps.

These parotid problems may last seven to ten days. The duration of the actual illness itself is variable but children tend to get off more lightly than adults. In a typical mild, uncomplicated case the glands swell over two to three days, the swelling subsiding seven to ten days later. There is usually fever which can last about five days. Chewing may be uncomfortable especially sharp and sour foods. The mouth feels dry because the glands do not produce their usual quota of saliva. Occasionally the other salivary glands under the chin swell up.

In more severe cases the first flu-like symptoms are worse. The child may complain of earache, headache, sore throat and have a fever around the 39.5°C mark. (A higher reading suggests complications.)

Fortunately, in childhood a complete recovery is the usual outcome.

Complications
These are not common. The most usual, and most feared and widely known, is swelling of one or (rarely) both of the testicles. This is very rare before puberty. It occurs after puberty in perhaps a quarter of the men who go down with mumps. Sterility is rare, but it makes good sense for young men to avoid contact with mumps if at all possible. This complication is one good reason for boys to get immunity to the mumps virus before puberty either by catching it or by vaccination.

Mumps can cause inflammation of the brain, as can other viral illnesses. The danger signs are headache, high fever, and stiff neck. Your doctor will obviously need to see the child if you are worried about this. However, these problems alarming as they are, usually settle quickly and completely.

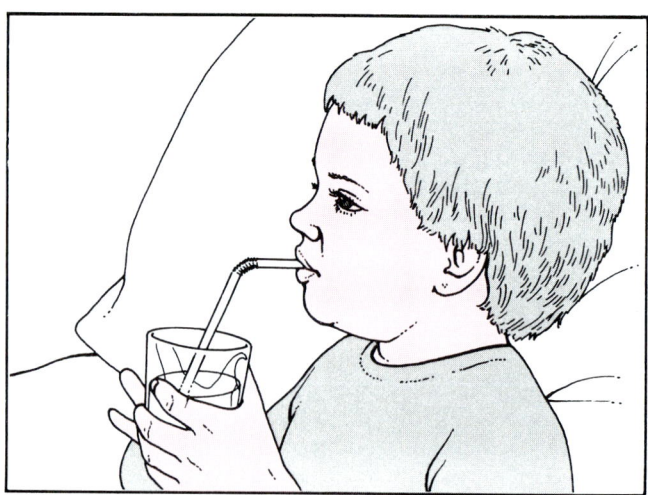

Opening the mouth is painful during a bad dose of mumps, but it is important that the mouth is kept moist. A child may find it more comfortable to drink using a straw. Avoid sharp flavoured drinks which make the parotid gland work overtime.

Treatment
The only treatment for mumps is to help relieve the symptoms while the child recovers. Let the child stay in bed if he or she doesn't feel like getting up. The mouth needs careful attention because opening it may be painful and the inside can be dry, so lots to drink, paracetamol in the correct dose, and perhaps a scarf around the neck for comfort.

Vaccination
A vaccine against mumps became available in the late 1960s. It has not been as widely used as some of the other vaccines, but is now available in the combined MMR vaccination (see pages 156-157). Once you have had mumps you are almost certainly immune for life.

Measles

Measles is one of the most infectious of the childhood illnesses and is caused by a virus. This virus spreads from person to person through the air in tiny droplets of moisture.

Signs and symptoms
The first signs are like that of a heavy cold. The eyes are sore and inflamed, the nose runny and the cough troublesome. The temperature is high. Sometimes the child seems much better for 24 hours, only to worsen again. Then comes the rash which is the main sign of a bout of measles. It comes two to four days after the cold symptoms have developed. It usually starts behind the child's ears and quickly spreads to the face. After this it appears on the trunk. By this time the child is probably feeling better. The rash lasts about five days.

With a little experience (and this book!) it becomes fairly easy to spot a case a measles: a miserable, blotchy red child, with red eyes and crusted nostrils, breathing through the mouth between coughs and sneezes. A diagnosis is clinched by seeing a tell-tale rash which looks like grains of salt on the insides of the cheeks just above the lower teeth at the back (Koplik's spots).

There is often a fever with measles and this may rise and fall before it goes completely. During the time the child is feverish there may be a cough which is often the last symptom to go.

Complications

The usual complication after catching measles is another infection on top of it. This is usually caused by a bacteria which invades either the ear or the lungs.

If the child deteriorates on the fourth day of the rash, then suspect something else has happened. Youngsters under two years are particularly at risk of this type of secondary infection, so if the fever does not abate, or after the third day of the rash the cough worsens, or the child has earache, call the doctor.

Antibiotics have no effect on viruses, so cannot be used to combat the measles germ itself. However, your doctor may prescribe antibiotics to clear up a secondary infection.

There are some other very rare complications; inflammation of the brain (meningitis) is one (it occurs once in every million cases). However, remember that ear problems are by far the most likely.

Treatment

There isn't any except to make your child feel as comfortable as possible until he or she recovers. The usual things apply; warms drinks, paracetamol to bring down the fever and ease aches and pains, and lots of tender loving care. If there is any eye discharge wash it away with cotton wool dipped in boiled water which has cooled. Use a fresh swab for each eye. There is no need to nurse in the dark unless that is what the child wants.

Vaccination

There is now an effective vaccine which can safely be given to most children. Measles is a very unpleasant illness. It can be prevented. Complications following the vaccine are ten times rarer than those following the natural disease. Measles is so infectious that almost all children will catch it if they have not been vaccinated.

Scarlet fever

Scarlet fever is an infection caused by a streptoccocal bacteria. It is distinguished from other similar throat infections by a distinctive red rash, hence the name. The germ that causes scarlet fever is killed by antibiotics, so penicillin (or one of the other antibiotics) will almost always combat the infection. Improved standards of hygiene and nutrition have made this disease very rare indeed.

Whooping cough

Whooping cough (also called pertussis) is a very infectious and dangerous illness caused by a bacteria.

Signs and symptoms

The main symptom is the cough. At first it is dry and hacking, and is likely to be the first sign that all is not well. A clear runny nose is also common during the early part of the illness. During this early stage (which lasts about a week) the child is not very ill, but is very infectious. However, it is not apparent yet that this is whooping cough because the characteristic whoop has not yet started.

When it does develop after about ten days it comes in spasms. During the spasm the child's face turns dark red, the eyes bulge, and the child eventually coughs up white sticky sputum. The most characteristic and punishing aspect of the cough is that it comes in bursts during the same breath. Normally a child would take a breath in before giving a cough out. (Try a cough now yourself — you take a breath without even having to think.) With whooping cough the coughs come so suddenly that the child has no chance to take air into the lungs. This is very distressing. After the burst of coughing is over the child whoops to get air quickly back into the lungs. This is a trick that older children develop. Babies may not whoop making the cough difficult to diagnose. It also makes the infection much more serious and distressing in young babies.

After a bout of coughing the child may be sick. He or she is often too weak to feed, and begins to loose weight. During this part of the illness these bouts may come every few minutes but over some weeks the coughing becomes gradually less severe. However, it is some months before patients lose their coughs and cease to be a worry. Some doctors warn parents that the cough may last 100 days.

Treatment

Antibiotics are believed to be effective against the bacteria which causes all this. The problem is that the medicine has to be given early before the germ damages the lungs. By the time the whoops come it is too late. It is not often possible to give them in time because during that first stage of the dry cough and runny nose, whooping cough may not be suspected. This means it is important to tell your doctor if an unprotected child is in contact with whooping cough.

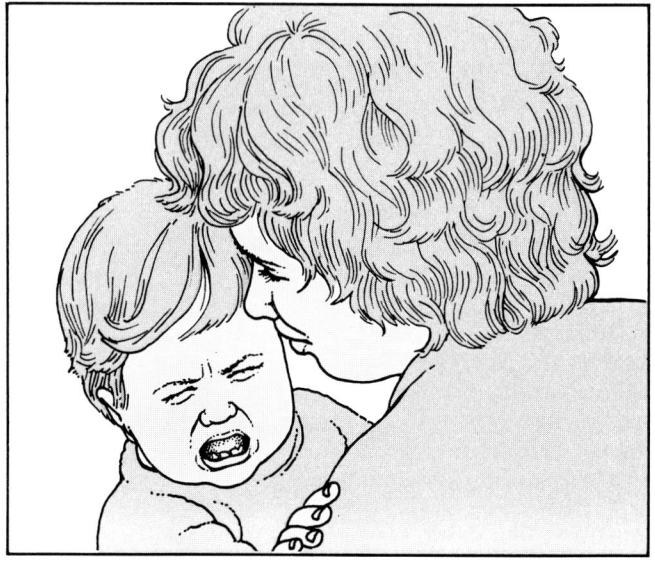

Whooping cough is very distressing in young babies. Cuddle and comfort the child during each bout.

Actual nursing care during the worst of the cough is a round-the-clock affair. If the child is very unwell, and it is young babies who are the worry, then it may be necessary to nurse them in the hospital.

The child will find it comforting to be held firmly and securely in your arms during the worst of the coughing spasms. During the coughing bouts it is often a good idea to turn the child's head down because this makes it easier to bring up the white plugs of sputum.

Feeding is often a problem. One ploy is to offer the child a small amount of food soon after he or she has been sick because it has a better chance of staying down.

Cough medicines are of no use during this distressing time. My advice is not to waste time and money on them. Whooping cough is a disease that your doctor must notify to the authorities. From this and all that has been said it is clearly an illness that needs professional help and guidance.

Complications
The common ones fall into three groups and again it must be emphasized that the age of the child is important. The younger the child, the worse the complications.

One major problem is physical damage to the lungs from all the coughing. Your doctor may want an X ray at some stage to check that the lungs are fully expanded with air. The other complication is related to this. Different bacteria may invade damaged lung tissue and cause pneumonia.

The ear is another part of the body which can suffer from a secondary infection. Antibiotics may need to be given to these children.

The third area of concern may be the vomiting which can lead not only to undernourishment, but also to the loss of important body fluids.

Prevention
Whooping cough can be prevented by vaccination. No one argues about this. The only reasons not to have your child vaccinated is if he or she, or any close relative has had fits or any kind of brain or nerve disorder. Take the advice of your doctor.

Whooping cough is very infectious and babies do not get any immunity from their mothers during the first months of life. This means that if these children are to be vaccinated the course of three injections should be started as early as is practical. This usually around three months, but can be earlier. It is important to keep an unvaccinated child out of contact with whooping cough.

If your child receives the full three injections against whooping cough there is about a one in five chance of getting a very mild attack of the disease. However, the majority of children are completely protected. The risks of whooping cough vaccination are very small. Your child is at least ten times more likely to get complications (like brain damage) from the natural disease than from the vaccine.

Roseola infantum
A mild viral illness with a rash mainly seen in children under three. It is very much like German measles, except that the rash of pink spots comes after the temperature has gone down.

Complications
Febrile convulsions are possible if the child has a high temperature.

Disease Incubation time	Rash	Appearance and disappearance of rash
Chickenpox 14-21 days	Red pimples which soon turn into blistery small spots. These burst easily. A crust forms in a few days. The spots come in crops. Scabs fall off leaving pink marks.	First sign of the illness. Spots come out over three days. Most will have crusted and fallen off after about ten days.
Measles 14-21 days	Dark red spots starting behind the ears which soon form large, irregular red blotches. Child feels better as rash and fever subside.	Rash appears about the fourth day of the illness and lasts about five days.
Mumps 14-21 days	No rash	———
Rubella 7-14 days	A light pink rash, often beginning on the face and neck and spreading to body. May even go unnoticed. Does not peel.	Comes when the child first feels ill and lasts only a few days.
Whooping cough 7-14 days	No rash	———

Child no longer infectious	Vaccination and immunity
From five days before the rash until all the spots have crusted and fallen off. Children with chickenpox cannot give adults shingles.	Healthy children need no kind of vaccination or immunity. One attack gives life-long immunity.
From when the child starts to feel ill until about four days after the rash appear (about eight days in total).	Protection from mother usually lasts for the first year of life. For this reason the MMR triple vaccination is usually delayed until the second year. A single dose of vaccine is thought to protect child for life.
Seven days after glands go down.	MMR triple vaccine given in injection form at fourteen months. A single dose of vaccine is thought to protect child for life.
About five days after the start of the rash.	MMR triple vaccine given in injection form at fourteen months. A single dose of vaccine is thought to protect child for life. However, if your daughter was born before the MMR vaccine became available, ask your doctor about her immunity before she reached puberty.
After about four weeks from when the first hacking cough started. This is about three weeks from the start of any whoop.	Vaccination prevents most children catching (and spreading) whooping cough. If it is caught after vaccination it will be mild. Remember, mothers do not give any immunity to their babies (unlike measles), so vaccination can start at three months or even before.

Meningitis

This is a serious condition where the membranes (meninges) covering the brain become inflamed. Get medical help immediately if you suspect it.

Suspect meningitis if several (but not necessarily all) of the following apply

- The child has a severe headache.
- The child has a fever, often over 39°C.
- The child dislikes bright light.
- The child has a stiff neck.
- The child vomits.
- The child becomes drowsy and confused.

Some cases of meningitis are accompanied by a red skin rash which is a blotchy red purple colour. It is caused by bleeding under the skin and does not fade if you press it. It can appear very quickly.

Signs in young babies
These are very difficult to detect, and of course the baby cannot tell you what is wrong. Babies with meningitis may have none of the typical symptoms you may see in older children. They may simply be listless, pasty looking, and off feeds.

This is not to say you should worry each time the baby is off colour that the problem is meningitis. However, have meningitis in the back of your mind if a child seems unusually unwell. It is not easy to detect even for experienced doctors, and so if in any doubt ask for help.

The most reliable sign of meningitis is that the mood of the baby or child suddenly changes for the worse. It is difficult to describe until you see this. Fortunately not many of you will see a child with meningitis. However, many parents who do for the first time instinctively know something serious is wrong even if they do not know what.

Meningitis often occurs in outbreaks and epidemics affect a community from time to time. Your doctor may prescribe antibiotics for anyone who has been in close contact with a case of meningitis. Only very occasionally is vaccination necessary.

Remember that although meningitis is a very frightening condition, most cases will get better without the need for antibiotics. In its mild form meningitis is one of the complications of mumps.

Stiff neck
Many of the feverish illnesses of childhood are accompanied by stiffness in the neck. This is usually mild and, although the child complains of aches, he or she is able to touch the chin onto the chest. This is not usually possible if the stiff neck is caused by meningitis. But remember, this is not the only criteria on which to judge if a child has meningitis. If you are worried, get the doctor to check.

Fevers

The normal body temperature of a child varies between 36°C and 37.5°C. It is important to realize that it very often varies during the day, often being a degree higher in the evening than it was in the morning.

Important!

A fever is not a particularly reliable way of judging if a child is really ill or not. The height of a fever is not related to the severity of an illness.

Very ill babies may not have a raised temperature whereas some children's temperatures can go up and down without any serious problems, so do not use a temperature as a reliable indicator. Your own judgement of the child's general state is a much better guide. Of course a fever may be one of your worries and if so, ring the doctor for advice.

Taking a child's temperature
There are a number of places to take a child's temperature, under the tongue, under the arm and inside the rectum (back passage).

A cooperative older child can have the temperature taken in the mouth or under the arm. It may seem an obvious thing to say but explain carefully to the child that if he or she bites the thermometer, it will break. If it breaks in the mouth the glass is a greater hazard than the mercury which in liquid form is harmless.

It is not safe to put a glass thermometer in a young child's mouth, but under the arm is a useful alternative. Remember that a temperature taken here will tend to be a degree lower than one taken in the mouth. Raise the child's arm, tuck the thermometer into the centre of the armpit, then cuddle the child holding the arm securely against his or her side.

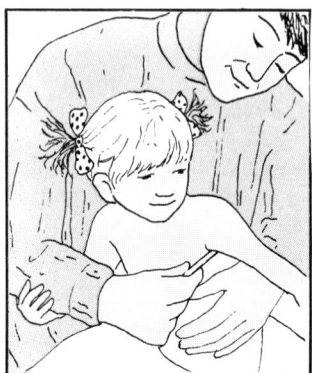

It is safer to take a young child's temperature under the arm. Strip thermometers are sometimes useful but can be inaccurate.

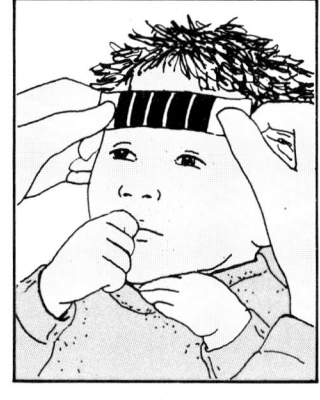

A temperature taken in the mouth will be a degree or two higher than one taken under the arm.

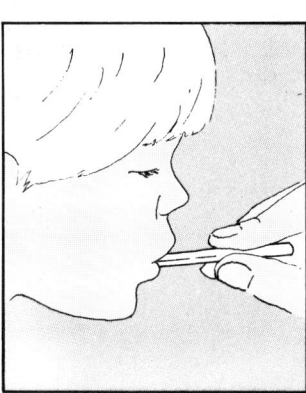

A common mistake when taking temperatures is to take the thermometer out too quickly. I would suggest you time at least two minutes on a clock or watch before reading the instrument. Also make sure that the bulb is in the right place. It is very easy to put the thermometer half-heartedly under the tongue and allow the child to breathe through the mouth giving a low reading.

Febrile convulsions

Some children under five have a tendency to fit if their temperature goes up. This does not happen to all children, and it very rarely happens after a child is five. It may run in families and it does not mean the child will go on to have epilepsy later in life. If one of your children has had a febrile convulsion, you should be on the alert with the others.

Signs and symptoms

A febrile convulsion is a very frightening thing to see. The whole episode is not unlike an epileptic fit. The child is unconscious and twitching and jerking. The teeth are tighly clenched, the eyes may be closed or you may see them roll. Often the child is incontinent and may go blue.

This stage lasts less than a few minutes. Lay him or her on one side in the recovery position (see page 147).

The fit in itself should not cause permanent harm even though it appears to be such an alarming event. After it is over the child will probably fall into a peaceful sleep.

Important!

● Do not force anything into the mouth.
● Stay with the child and do not allow anything to block the airway. The best position is to lay the child on one side.
● Stop the child's body coming to any harm during the jerking stage. This does not mean it is necessary to restrain by force. The child is unconscious and you should stay calm and guide him or her into a comfortable safe position.
● Cool the child off when the crisis is over and get help from the doctor.

Prevention

As always, this is better than cure. A hot child needs to be cooled and the old practice of keeping a feverish child wrapped up in blankets next to a fire just pushes the temperature higher. It needs to come down. If the temperature goes above 38.8°C then sponge the skin down with tepid water, and continue to give the paracetamol elixir which you will probably have been using since the child was first feverish.

The child must obviously be comfortable, so do not sit them outside in a winter garden! But you could open the bedroom window, and take off any extra layers of clothes. Give lots to drink to replace fluid lost in sweat.

°F	96	97	98	99	100	101	102	103	104
°C	35.6	36.1	36.7	37.2	37.8	38.3	38.9	39.4	40

Call the doctor if:
● You are worried and want help or advice. This is a very important reason.
● The temperature keeps going up despite efforts to get it down, particularly if the child has had a febrile convulsion before.
● The child develops symptoms such as a headache with vomiting, dislike of light, and drowsiness because these may be signs of meningitis, an inflammation of the covering of the brain. A baby may be off feeds, lethargic and irritable.
● The child seems unusually unwell. This ties in with the first reason for calling the doctor. It may seem a rather vague statement to put into a book that you have turned to for answers, but parents are very good at knowing when something is really wrong with their child. They may not know the long names for illnesses. But they know when their child is not getting better.

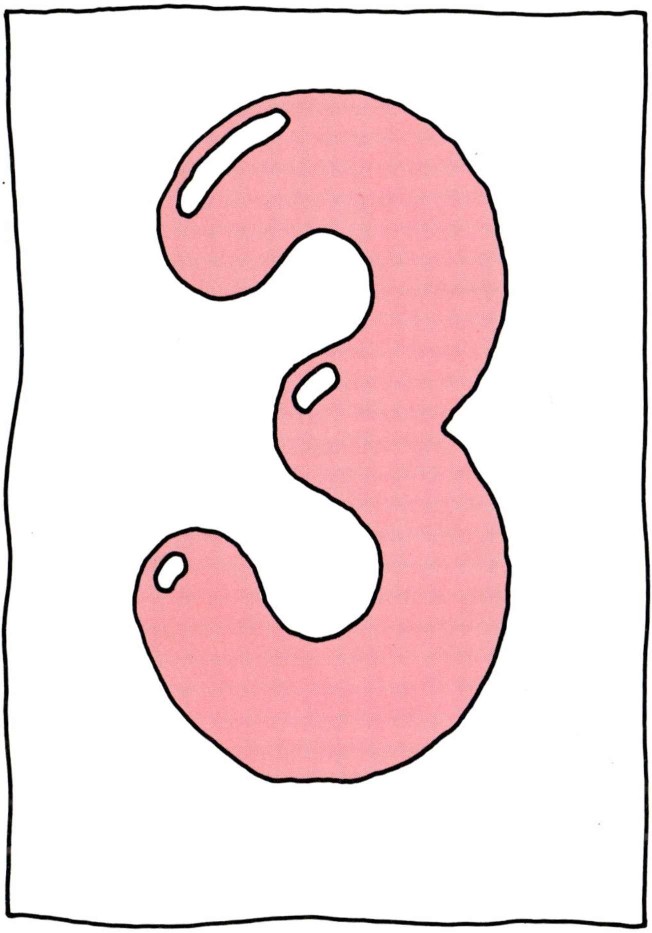

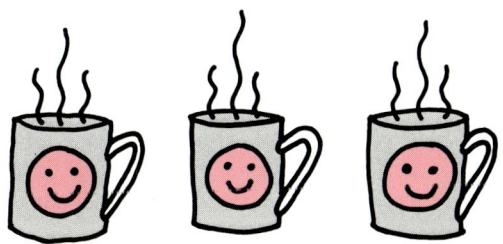

Coughs and colds

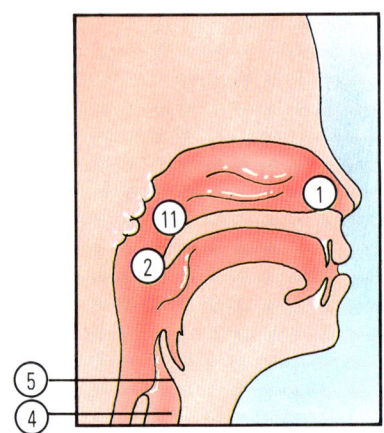

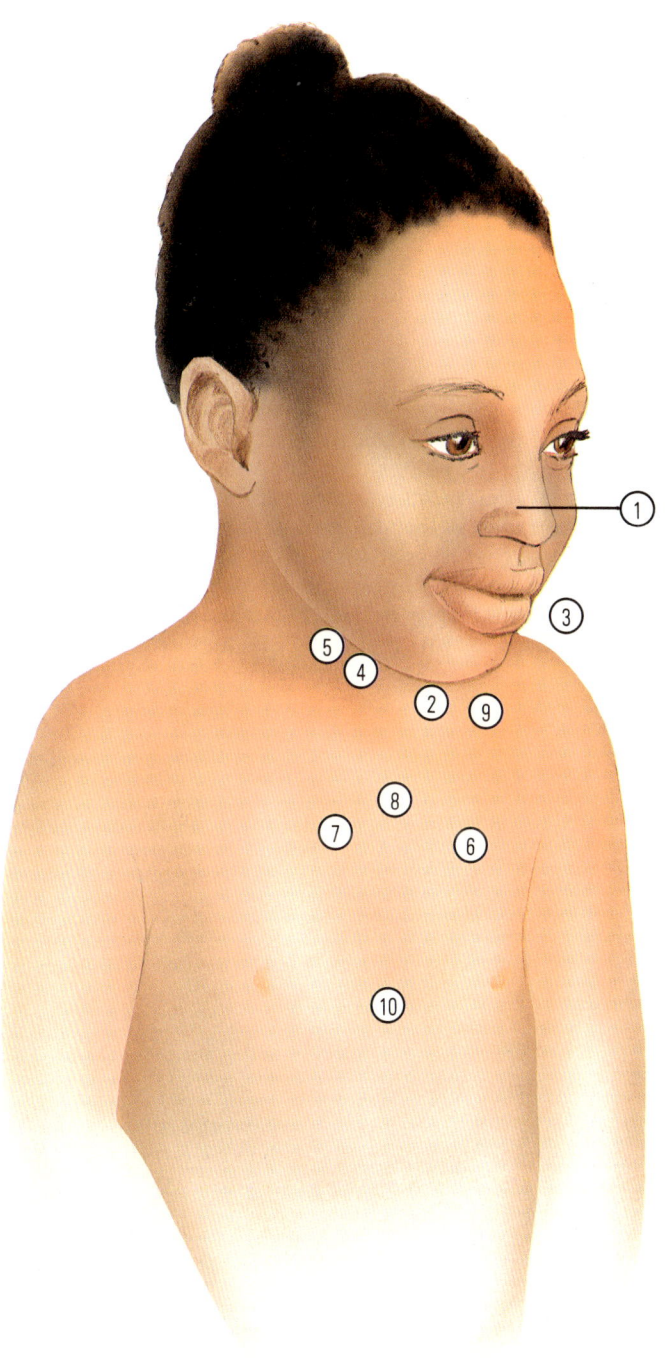

Coughs and colds

A normal child will have between six and twelve colds every year. There's not very much you or the doctor can do to change this fact of young life! It helps, however, if you can understand what is going on and, more importantly, recognize the complications that can develop and which require your doctor's help.

A cold is an infection caused by a virus. There are probably hundreds of different cold viruses that do this. It is hardly ever necessary to find out exactly which one is responsible because it does not make any difference to the treatment.

Antibiotics have no effect on viruses and are useless in the treatment of uncomplicated colds. Because the variety and number of viruses are constantly changing it is impossible to make an effective vaccine.

The virus attacks the upper air passages. Symptoms start about one to four days after the virus has been breathed in. It gets into the cells lining the air passages and triggers them into producing excessive mucus. The nose runs, catarrh drips down the back of a sore throat and accumulates as mucus which needs to be coughed up. Generally the child is miserable, achey, feels bunged up and is in need of some tender loving care. These symptoms may vary a little from person to person and from cold to cold.

The cough that accompanies a cold is a good thing. It protects the child's lungs by bringing up phlegm.

After a few days the clear mucus running out of the nose may change colour. After the initial sneezing stage the problem tends to be the sticky, yellowish catarrh which needs blowing away. The cold symptoms then subside — at least until the next one comes along!

Home nursing

While the symptoms are at their worst the child should be nursed at home. It is probably kinder to everyone to keep those with a real streamer off school. They are best looked after quietly at home in the warm with plenty of their favourite fruit drinks.

A blocked nose can be more difficult to tackle. Very young babies should be laid down on their sides without a pillow because this helps prevent catarrh running down the back of the throat which makes them cough. Before the age of about four to six months children can become very upset by a blocked nose. This becomes especially obvious when they are trying to feed from a bottle or at the breast. They have not yet learnt to cope with breathing temporarily through the mouth and feeding. They feel unable to breathe and the result is often a coughing, spluttering young baby who appears very distressed indeed.

This is where decongestants have a role to play. They can be given in the prescribed dose just before a feed which helps to avoid this choking. Nose drops can also be used just before the baby is put down for a sleep. Only use these for two to three days as they can cause congestion if used for too long. Older children may be helped by some of the over-the-counter medicines but usually the best way to deal with a stuffed and blocked nose is simply to encourage the child to sit up and blow the nose clear.

Teach the older child to gently blow one nostril at a time. This helps protect the nasal passages. It is a mistake to blow hard with both nostrils blocked. This can force germ laden air into the ear.

Treatment

Paracetamol is useful for general flu-like symptoms and also helps to relieve most of the aches and any soreness in the throat. Paracetamol is a very good mild pain killer and will not cause any stomach upset. Aspirin is not recommended for children because of possible very rare side effects. In its basic form most children (and adults — try it yourself!) find paracetamol unpleasant to taste. There are various preparations for children (Calpol, Calpol Six plus, Panadol junior, and Disprol) which taste nicer. Follow the instructions and there will be no problems. Your child may develop a preference for one particular brand or another.

Decongestants

Most of these come as either sprays or drops and make the blood vessels lining the nose constrict which reduces the swelling. It is important not to use them too often as the effect is only temporary, and long term use (for longer than three weeks) reduces their effectiveness and may even make the runny nose worse. The two most popular preparations are ephedrine and xylometazoline 0.05% (Otrovine Paediatric).

Antihistamines
These drugs are often used in cold treatments but they are an unpredictable group of drugs and must be used with care as some will make a child excitable rather than sleepy. Find one which suits your child by striking a balance between sedation (very useful at night for coughs) and drying up a runny nose. Apart from their sedative effect, they are only of use when the symptoms are due to an allergy.

It is impossible for a book to give precise advice on antihistamines for other people's children. Use them sparingly and with caution. I give my own children ones like trimeprazine (Vallergan) or promethazine (Phenergan) at night which sedates the child, supresses any cough, and gives everyone a good night's sleep. They are well tried, trusty and safe.

Prevention

Prevention is the best policy, especially with colds which have no cure. Remind children that coughs and sneezes really do spread diseases. Strict quarantine is impractical with such a common illness that is not going to cause a healthy child any lasting harm. (If we did isolate our children they would hardly see one another during the winter!) The one exception is with very young babies. People with colds should be kept away from them if at all possible. A person with a cold is infectious to others for 24

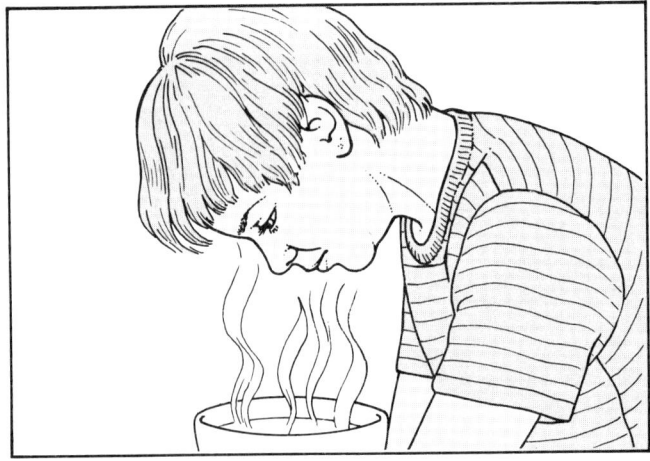

An inhalation before bed greatly relieves cold congestion.

hours before the symptoms first develop until the cold has been going for about five days.

It is probably because colds are so common and annoying that they attract more than their share of myths and useless home remedies. It is scientifically proven, for example, that colds are not caused by getting cold. A child is not going to catch a cold by playing outside with wet socks, or going to school without a scarf.

Colds are, however, much more common in winter as this is when cold viruses strike. Windows are likely to be shut at school and central heating circulates the air, all of which helps the cold virus to spread.

Another myth relates to diet. If a child is eating a well-balanced diet there is no need for vitamin supplements or tonics as these will not stop children catching one cold after another. In particular, there is no evidence that large doses of vitamin C prevent colds.

Most colds do not have complications. Only those who suffer from asthma or who have had ear, sinus or chest problems in the past may need to see the doctor for treatment. You will soon learn whether your child is prone to complications with a cold and recognize when to seek medical help. These patients may need antibiotics to fight bacteria. Do remember though that straight colds are caused by viruses and antibiotics do not work against these.

A cold is the most common illness in children. One advantage of this is that most people know one when they see one! There are a few other conditions, however, which can seem to be a simple cold when they are not so beware if things do not seem quite right. A one-sided nasal discharge, for example, could be the result of something stuck up the nose. A continual cold may be the result of an allergy of the upper air passages (see page 58).

Remember the doctor is there to help you if you are at all worried.

Call the doctor if:

● The child seems to get steadily worse.
● The child develops a high fever. Remember, an uncomplicated cold is not usually accompanied by a fever over 38°C.
● The clear mucus, wherever it is coming from, turns yellow or green.
● Earache develops.

Cough

A cough is a chest movement controlled by nerves and performed by muscles. A breath is taken in and the cough starts when an effort is made to breathe out. Pressure builds up because the airway is temporarily closed by the glottis. This is a flap at the top of the throat. When the glottis opens air shoots out very fast as a cough.

All this happens quickly and is instinctive. The purpose of a cough is to get rid of something irritating the lungs and it is a very useful and necessary reflex. Just think how quickly children cough (often called choking or gagging) when food goes down the wrong way.

So how do you know if a cough is serious? The answer is that you don't until you know what the cause is.

Common causes

These are arranged in descending order according to where the trouble arises. It is helpful to know that when -itis is tagged onto the name of part of the body it means that that part is inflamed.

Post nasal drip

This is a chronic infection or allergy, probably starting with a viral infection, in which lots of mucus and catarrh drips down to irritate the lungs from areas of tonsillitis, adenoiditis, rhinitis, and sinusitis. The end result is a cough. Post-nasal drip is by far and away the commonest cause of a cough.

Laryngitis

This is usually the result of a virus and causes a sore throat, some voice changes (it becomes hoarse but quiet!) and a dry cough. Little treatment is needed other than the general measures we have discussed. Warm wet air helps the most so try inhalations with menthol or eucalyptus first.

Croup

(The medical name for this is laryngotracheobronch-itis!) Croup is caused by inflammation of the vocal cords and the main windpipe which carries air down to the lungs. It may follow a cold when the virus spreads to the windpipe or, rarely, by bacteria infecting a little flap in the throat called the epiglottis.

Children affected by croup are usually between the ages

of six months and about three years. The younger the child the more serious it is because a small tube narrows proportionately more than a larger one does. It is uncommon after five years and very rare in children older than seven.

Two main symptoms are a harsh cough and difficulty in breathing. Very often they have had a cold and gone to bed fairly well but a sudden attack of croup wakes them up. Subsequent attacks usually occur at night.

The cough is one which once heard is never forgotten. It is like a high pitched throaty bark. Breathing is a struggle with a growling noise on breathing in. Very often the chest wall is drawn in with the strain of this. Understandably the children are often frightened and struggling for air. At this stage the main symptom is shortness of breath.

Call the doctor if:

- You are at all worried
- The child's face becomes blue
- The child is fighting for breath

Children occasionally die from croup if it is not relieved, so if you are in any doubt about the health of a child with symptoms like this, call the doctor.

Home nursing

The most important point to remember when dealing with a sick child is that your calm presence and reassurance is a great comfort, especially as these children are understandably panicky. Never leave a child with croup alone. If necessary, one adult should stay up all night with the child but this situation justifies a call to the doctor.

Dry, warm air seems to make the croup worse. As a parent, the best practical help you can give is to improve the air in the sick room. Open the window for a while if your house is centrally heated or boil a kettle in the room to create a warm, humid atmosphere. Never leave a child unsupervised with a boiling kettle or set it too close to him or her where it might scald or burn. For fast relief run a hot, steamy bath, take the child into the bathroom and keep the door shut to build up the steam. Alternatively, fill the kitchen with steam by putting boiling saucepans on all rings of the cooker. Cuddle the child in his or her most comfortable position.

A dry cough and hoarse voice is often produced by an ordinary cold. The doctor is not needed but an extra pillow and a warm room should make the patient more comfortable.

Chest infections

These include bronchitis which is an inflammation of the bronchi (main lung airways) and pneumonia which is a lung infection. It is often difficult to separate the two as the symptoms are much the same. A chest infection leads to a distressed, hot, ill child with breathing noises that sound like a broken accordion. All sorts of wheezing, grunting and hacking noises are made by the chest.

Children suffering like this will probably need to see the doctor when he is on his rounds. If the condition rapidly goes from bad to worse with the child becoming frighteningly short of breath or confused and disorientated, call him or her straight away. Antibiotics may be necessary, as well as the treatments for cough and fever which we have already talked about. Modern antibiotics have saved the lives of thousands of these children. Most will not even have to go into hospital, but recovery may take a week or two. As with other illnesses, kindness and general nursing care will be a great comfort to the child.

As children do not smoke, chronic problems are rare. Chest problems are worse, however, in children who spend time with smokers. Try to prevent sufferers from coming into contact with cigarette smoke. Remember the younger the child the more serious this sort of illness can be. After about the age of eight these sorts of infection become much less frequent.

Asthma

This chest condition is usually easily recognized once you have heard it a few times. The basic wheezy, whistling noise comes when air is breathed out. Asthma and allergies are discussed in full in Chapter 4. If the attack is the basis of a cough, make a mental note as to when it occurs such as going to bed or running at games. Tell your doctor if you think the cough can be linked to a particular place, time or activity.

Your doctor is the best person to advise you if any extra medicine is necessary during these attacks. It is important not to give the child the notion that he or she has an illness which in some way will make for a life of chronic bad health and restriction. Nowadays asthmatics can lead full lives taking part in all sports and activities.

Measles or whooping cough

Both of these infectious diseases cause coughing. They are dealt with in full in Chapter 2.

Whooping cough is in a league of its own. During the early dry cough and runny nose stage, whooping cough may not be suspected so it is important to tell your doctor if an unprotected child has been in contact with it.

Inhaled foreign body

This should always be taken seriously. Try and stop children running about with sweets and other sorts of food in their mouths. Take the same view towards small toys being carried in the mouth. It would not take much for the foreign body to find its way into the child's air passages if he or she were to fall or be knocked accidentally (see Choking, page 134).

If the foreign object is small it is likely to have gone further down into the lungs and lodged in one of the air passages. Once this happens it will have to be removed through an instrument which is passed into the mouth and

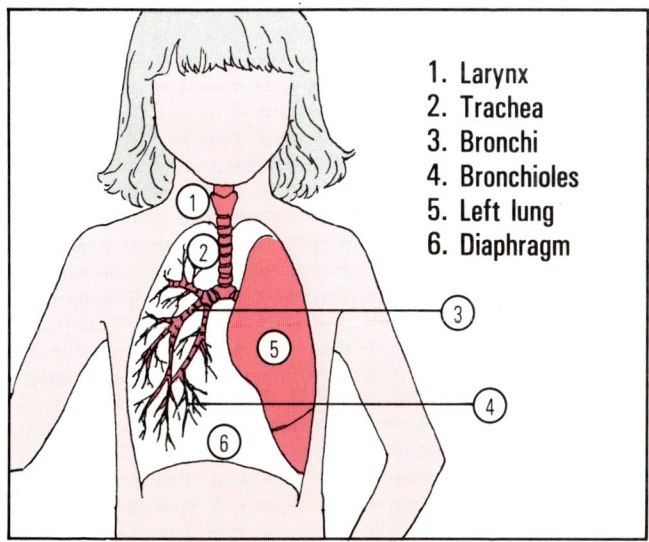

1. Larynx
2. Trachea
3. Bronchi
4. Bronchioles
5. Left lung
6. Diaphragm

down the windpipe by a surgeon. (No cutting into the chest is necessary.)

One of the most common things that a child can inhale is a peanut and it is in fact one of the most dangerous. If removed quickly there is little trouble but complications develop when the peanut gets into the lungs and goes unnoticed. Severe infections can then occur. Less toxic objects like beads can lie undetected in the lungs for weeks, but peanuts and foods like a piece of bone or a crumb can quickly produce a nasty pneumonia or even an abscess. Some doctors say that it is inadvisable to have peanuts in a home where there are children under three. Older children (and adults) should be discouraged from the party trick of throwing peanuts up into the air and catching them in their mouths. The nut can go down into the lung instead of the stomach without you realizing it.

Words like dry, tickly, fruity, barking, hacking, chesty and irritating are often used to describe coughs. They are not exact terms and I have been trying to understand them for years. This is what I think they mean:
● dry and tickly — when there is no mucus
● chesty and fruity — when there is mucus on the chest
● barking — when the larynx (or voice box) is inflamed
● irritating — when mucus is dripping into the lungs or when the rest of the family are being kept awake!

If you end up only slightly confused by these descriptions then you have done well!

Cough medicines

These are of very limited value in treating children despite the fact that there are so many available. Many are sold as cold treatments and contain a mixture of various drugs. Cough treatments in general have two effects. They either suppress a cough or they make sputum less sticky and easier to cough up.

Suppressants
There are some very good drugs which will stop a cough. The problem is that coughing is very often a useful reflex for children with colds as it keeps phlegm off the chest. Having said that there are coughs which are dry and serve no useful purpose; the barking cough which accompanies laryngitis is an example. Hot lemon drinks are more helpful here.

Codeine is a very effective cough suppressant and is used widely in adults. You will find it offered in cough medicines. Remember though that cough suppression usually does not make sense.

The use of antihistamines (see page 46) at night is probably the best form of treatment when treatment is necessary because they give some rest from the cough.

Expectorants
In theory these are a great idea. They work by irritating the lining of the stomach and making more sputum in the lungs. This extra sputum is more watery and easier to cough up. The trouble is that the dose necessary to do this can cause stomach pain.

Inhalations help older children to bring up phlegm. Menthol type preparations (Karvol capsules, Friars Balsam) added to hot water produce vapours which when inhaled in deep breaths for up to five minutes, help to relieve the symptoms, especially when taken just before bedtime.

However, favourite drinks and foods can have just as good an effect on a sick child as some of the shop bought medications.

With most coughs and colds the greatest help and comfort comes from Mum and Dad's reassurance. Children respond very well to this and it has the advantage that although priceless it is free.

Sore throat

Sore throats often seem a permanent feature in some young families! They are most common between the ages of four and eight and occur frequently throughout the year, though it is a condition which normal, healthy children grow out of.

Sore throats go hand in hand with many of the common childhood illnesses and are often the first sign that something is wrong. Young children especially find it hard to describe what is making them feel unwell. A sore throat is an easy problem for them to describe.

Most are caused by viruses and only need paracetamol to relieve the pain. They last two or three days and then clear up on their own. Gargles are of little use as tests have shown that gargling does not reach back far enough into the throat. Like all safe methods of treatment, however, use them if they make your child feel better.

Call the doctor if:

● After three or four days the child does not appear to be getting any better, especially if his or her general health appears to be worsening.

● The child's temperature goes up above 38.3°C.

● An earache or headache, neck stiffness and vomiting develops.

Tonsils and adenoids

These are made of lymphatic material and form part of the body's natural defence mechanism. They are linked to a protective chain of glands in the throat and neck and are sited like soldiers at the gates to fight unwelcome germs as they enter the body through the mouth and nose.

You can see the two tonsils on each side of the back of the throat. The thing hanging down at the back of your mouth is not a tonsil but your uvula. The adenoids are out of sight behind the nose on the back wall of the pharynx. The other lymph glands in the neck are not usually possible to feel until they enlarge.

Tonsils and adenoids start to get smaller after the age of about seven. This is because infectious diseases become less common as the child gets older and they are not needed as much.

Before that they can take up a lot of space. When you look at some children's tonsils you wonder how on earth food gets by! But it nearly always does and size, suprisingly, is not that good an indicator of any likely problems.

The adenoids may take up a lot of the space in the back of the pharynx. This can force a child into breathing solely through the mouth which makes him or her sound nasal and will probably cause snoring.

Acute tonsillitis

This is most common in children under about nine. It is spread by droplets and is usually caused either by a bacteria (which penicillin will kill) or by a virus. It is not possible to tell by looking at the tonsils if they are infected by a virus or a bacteria.

Signs and symptoms

The child feels unwell, goes off his or her food, and finds swallowing painful. Complaints may be made about a sore

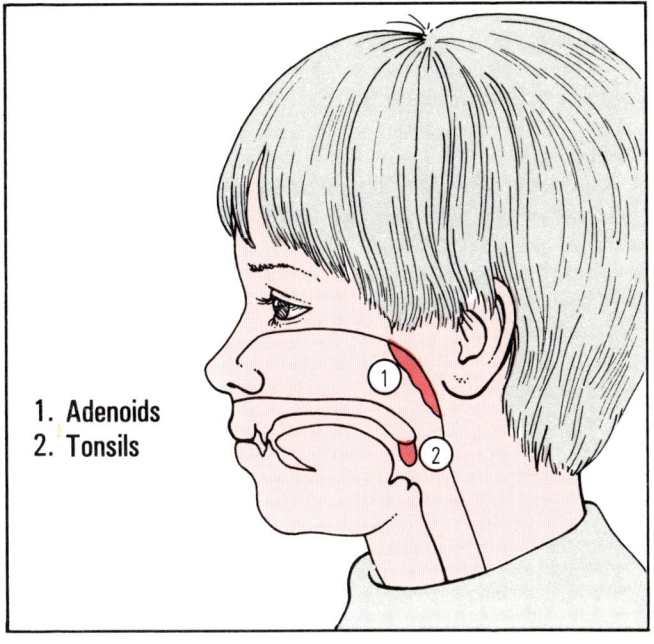

1. Adenoids
2. Tonsils

throat although, strangely, a young child with tonsillitis may say nothing about this. He or she may, however, complain of earache, stomach ache and headache.

The child appears hot and flushed and the lymph glands on the neck may be enlarged. Looking down the throat the tonsils will resemble large, red strawberries with streaks or spots of white.

The most common complication is a spread of the infection to the ear (see Chapter 4).

Treatment
The child needs to see the doctor who will probably prescribe an antibiotic if it seems a bacteria is involved.

Give the child the usual nursing care at home in the warm with plenty of rest and lots to drink with paracetamol mixtures. Do not let the child get too hot because of the risk of febrile convulsions. (See page 38).

Tonsillectomy and adenoidectomy (T and As)
You might well wonder why troublesome tonsils are not removed surgically straight away. It is important to understand that they are a useful and protective part of the

young body and worth keeping if at all possible. Sometimes, however, they are obviously having a limited effect and their removal is recommended. There are arguments for and against this operation.

Advantages
● Children who get repeated attacks are often much better after the operation although not always.
● They miss less school.
● Breathing is normal and general health improved.
● They will probably get fewer ear infections which reduce hearing.

Disadvantages
● No operation is without risk.
● Natural body defences are removed.
● Possibility of more bronchitis when older.
● Tonsillitis and earache will probably stop by the time children are nine even without an operation.

So what is the answer? Each child should be judged individually. Your doctor will advise and may well ask an ear, nose and throat specialist to give an opinion but if antibiotics (which are safe drugs) clear the attacks each time, why resort to surgery?

If the child keeps getting bouts of tonsillitis and it is obvious that the tonsils are unhealthy and not doing their job then removal may be considered. (The adenoids will probably be taken out at the same time.) This operation is rarely performed on a child under four as the situation will not have had time to develop.

If, however, a child is getting older and the attacks are getting less frequent then antibiotics should manage to hold the situation in check until the tonsils and adenoids shrivel up with age and become less prone to infection.

The most important consideration is the child's general health. The decision should not be swayed by the appearance of the tonsils.

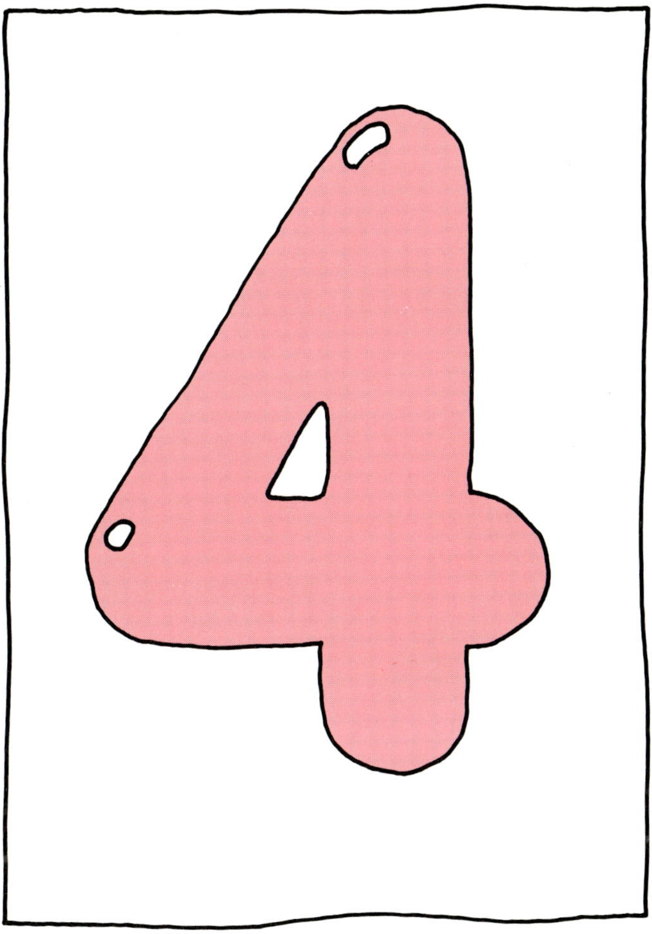

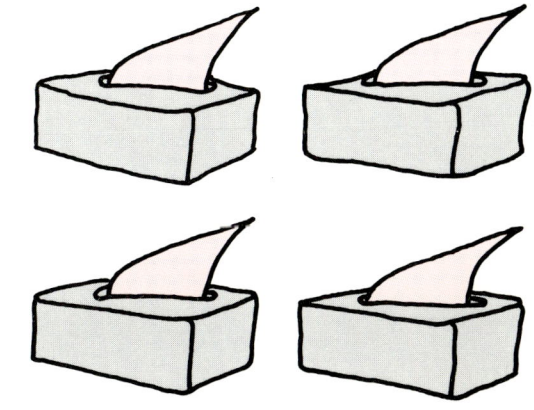

Allergies

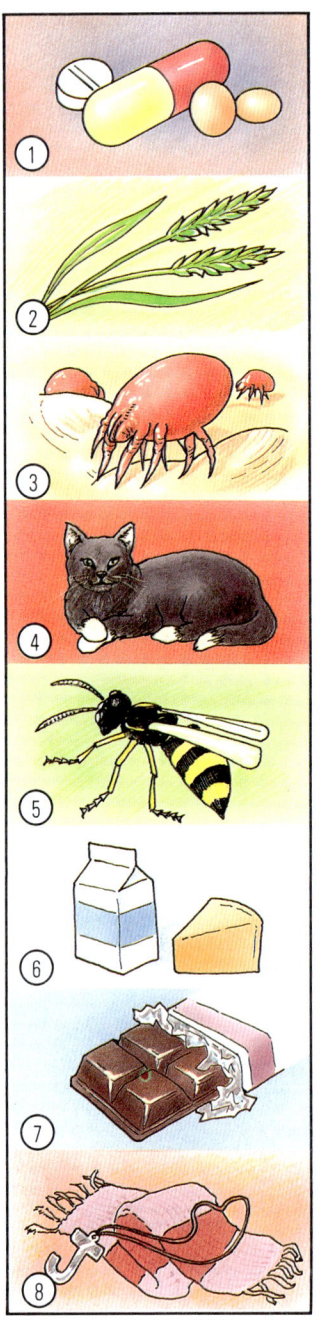

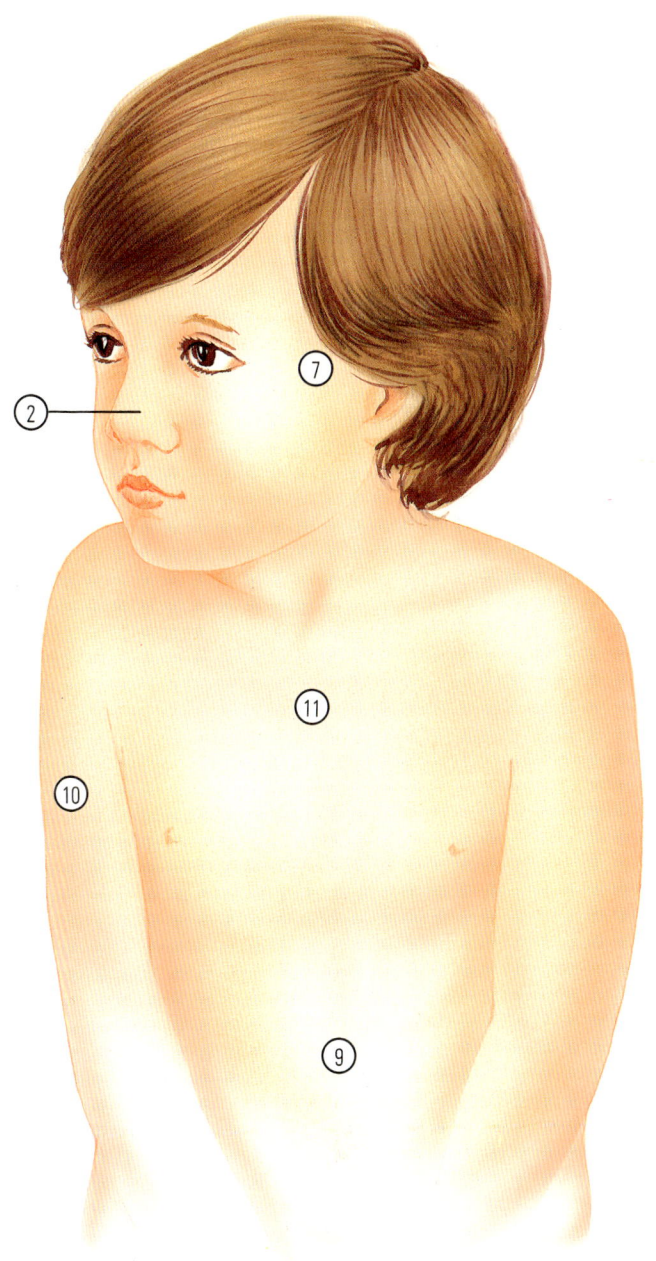

Allergies

An allergy is an over-reaction by the body a substance (usually a protein) which is called an allergen. The human body is continually exposed to potential allergens in the foods and drugs that we swallow, germs and pollen we breathe and plants, metals and chemicals that we touch.

The body protects itself from the outside world through the immune system, for example, by producing antibodies to fight off viruses. In the case of an allergy, however, the body reacts unnecessarily. This is an allergic reaction. It occurs for any number of reasons and has a variety of symptoms.

A great deal of research has gone into finding out about allergies and allergens, and there is still a lot to be learnt. A condition such as hay fever is clearly the result of an allergy, but many allergic reactions are probably not recognized for what they are. By the same token it is unhelpful to attribute every problem without an obvious cause to an allergy.

It has been estimated that one child in five suffers from allergic problems and the figure may be higher. A child may be allergic to a number of things which makes identifying the cause especially difficult.

Common allergic symptoms

Eyes and nose

Hay fever
Seasonal runny nose, puffy and runny eyes and sneezing. In this condition the problem is caused by allergens which are around at particular times of the year.

Perennial allergic rhinitis
In this condition the symptoms are caused by allergens present all year round.

When to suspect an allergy

Allergies tend to run in families, so if either parent, or a brother or sister suffer from something like hay fever, asthma or eczema, a child with the symptoms shown on the table may have an allergy.

The link between symptoms and allergens is often obvious, for example, if your child gets runny eyes, sneezes and a streaming nose whenever he or she plays with the neighbours' cat, the connection is not difficult to make. Other allergens may be harder to identify and will require some detective work. Keep a diary of the occurrence of symptoms. You may find that the role of seasonal factors, or particular places or stresses, becomes more obvious.

If straightforward remedies for a particular symptom do not work, the child may have an allergy. A good example of this is a persistent night-time cough which is not helped by courses of antibiotics. The problem is not an infection, but a reaction to something in the bedroom such as feather pillows or house dust mite. Although the child does not seem to wheeze, he or she may respond to asthma treatment.

Lungs

Asthma
Tight, wheezy chest because of narrowed airways and extra mucus production.

Intestines

Coeliac disease
In this gut allergy the small intestine reacts to gluten (a component of wheat flour) in the diet. There are probably many other food allergies producing symptoms such as tummy ache and diarrhoea.

Skin

Eczema (see Chapter 7)
Nettle rash (hives)
Papular urticaria

Finding the cause

The doctor can perform a skin test in which a small quantity of an allergen is pricked under the skin to see if it provokes a reaction. In theory the test sounds helpful in the identification of allergies but in practice it tends to be unreliable. Very often the results are inconclusive as what provokes a reaction during testing does not always have the same effect in everyday life. In some rare cases skin-testing causes a major reaction which is actually life-threatening.

For these reasons and because the child's immune system is underdeveloped and changing all the time the doctor will probably not recommend skin testing. It cannot be emphasized enough that the main way to find out what the child is allergic to is to carefully watch and see what provokes the allergy in the first place.

Hay fever

This common allergy is a reaction to grass pollens carried in the air in the summer months of June and July. Hay fever is, however, a term which describes more than a reaction to grasses. Tree pollens from as early as March and moulds as late as September can cause hay fever symptoms. Suspect hay fever when a cold seems to last all summer.

It is possible to predict when hay fever symptoms are likely to strike. This is useful when planning holidays, in assessing how the problem may affect schooling and in the timing of treatment.

Predicting hay fever attacks
● Even if the exact cause of the hay fever is not known, expect the symptoms at the same time each year and make allowances for late summers etc.
● Watch the weather. A wet spring will encourage grass growth and the summer pollen count is likely to be high. Wet days in the summer, however, keep the pollen count down. In June and July hot windy dry days cause most trouble.
● Take account of the area of the country in which you live. The true hay fever season is a week or two later in the North of England and Scotland than in London. Beware of pollen counts which may be taken hundreds of miles away and as much as 24 hours before.

Minimizing attacks
● Try and go away to the seaside during the worst of the season. Sea breezes tend to be free of grass pollens.
● If possible, keep car and house windows shut during June and July and when the child is outdoors sunglasses may be helpful.
● Avoid grassy areas. Keep the child indoors when the lawn is being mowed, and out of the countryside as far as is practical, particularly in the evening when pollens are descending with the cool air.
● Make sure teachers are aware of your child's difficulties as with goodwill there is much the school can do to help avoid attacks. An understanding with the school is important because as the child gets older hay fever may disrupt important school work and exams.

Medical treatment

Antihistamines
These medicines are taken by mouth and damp down the symptoms. Two of the more recent ones (Triludan and Hismanal) do not cause sleepiness but are not recommended for children under six. They take several days to achieve peak effectiveness.

Sodium Cromoglycate
This is the chemical name for a drug which comes in various forms for different parts of the body: Intal for lungs; Rynacrom for nose; and Opticrom for eyes.
    This drug is very free of side effects. It works by locking the stable door before the horse bolts. It does not produce instant relief, but is eventually so effective that there is a tendency to stop taking it in the belief that the problem is cured. Children should be strongly encouraged to keep up the treatment throughout the time they are exposed to the cause of the allergy. This is often all the year round, although for some the dose can be reduced say, in the winter.

Steroids
The doctor can prescribe these in various forms. Use them strictly as instructed.

Desensitization
Desensitizing injections work by introducing an allergen into the body so that the immune system learns not to

overreact when that allergen turns up in real life. You will need to discuss with your doctor if these might help your child but, like skin tests, they are rarely prescribed nowadays.

Do not despair with hay fever. There may not be a cure but children can be helped by the newer medicines, and many grow out of the problem.

House dust mite

This eight-legged beast lives in everyone's mattress and feeds off the scales shed from human skin. Unless you live in a mountainous area (the house dust mite does not like living above about 10,000 feet) then your bed is likely to be home to about 10,000! They are the cause of a lot of allergic symptoms such as wheezing, coughing and sneezing in the bedroom. The medical treatment is the same as for other similar allergic reactions (see Hay fever above).

It is possible, however, to reduce the population of mites in the bedroom with vigorous housework. This is far more effective than any medicine and can bring a dramatic relief of symptoms.

Reducing house dust mites
● Vacuum the mattress and cover it with polythene leaving one end open so that it can breathe. Wipe this polythene cover weekly and remove the cover monthly to vacuum the mattress. This will get rid of many of the mites and their food. A foam mattress probably does not need covering.
● Avoid nylon sheets which attract dust.
● Feather pillows and duvets are best replaced by synthetic materials. Avoid any kind of covers which collect dust. Use polyester-filled duvets instead.
● Cotton cellular blankets are much better than heavy feather duvets or eiderdowns. In general the less heavy the furnishing in the room the better.
● Damp dust the bedroom daily and the rest of the house if possible. Avoid brushing furniture and carpets.
● House dust mites like warm damp surroundings. Keep the house as dry and warm as possible. Avoid paraffin heaters which create a warm damp atmosphere.

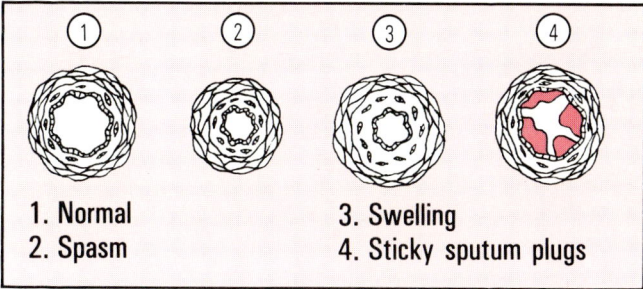

1. Normal
2. Spasm
3. Swelling
4. Sticky sputum plugs

Breathing difficulties occur when an asthma attack narrows the tiny muscular tubes in the lungs. This narrowing is caused by a number of things. The muscles themselves can go into a spasm and the delicate tube lining swells. Plugs of sputum accumulate and because breathing out is difficult the tubes are squeezed flat by pressure in the chest.

Asthma

Children with asthma have difficulty in breathing. This is the result of a narrowing of the small airways in the lung which also become clogged by sticky mucus. Asthma tends to run in families, and the child may be suffering from other allergic symptoms such as eczema and hay fever. Asthma rarely starts before the first year of life but if the child is going to suffer, he or she will almost certainly experience a first attack before the age of five. One child in ten will be affected at some stage though fortunately half will completely grow out of the tendency.

The causes fall into three main groups and often one or more factors are needed at the same time to trigger an attack.
1. Allergy
2. Infection
3. Emotional factors

Signs of an attack
An attack may start suddenly. The child is wheezy and has difficulty breathing, particularly breathing air out of the lungs. There may be a cough which is dry at first but then the child may bring up white plugs of sputum and complain that the chest feels tight.

It is important not to underestimate the severity of an asthma attack as the condition can suddenly deteriorate. Always call the doctor if you are worried, or the child does not respond to prescribed treatment.

Call the doctor IMMEDIATELY if:

● The wheeze gets worse and the child becomes distressed and struggles for air.
● The lips are blue because of lack of oxygen.
● The child is unable to talk because of the effort of breathing or is unable to complete a sentence without taking a breath. (Although I hope you never see a child as sick as this, it is a reliable warning sign of a bad attack and is easy for a non-medical person to detect.)
● The child is using extra muscles to breathe such as those around the neck and shoulders, and the tummy muscles. The abdomen may be drawn in to assist breathing.
● The child leans forward on elbows and won't lift them off the table or bed without becoming very distressed.

What to do until help arrives
Anxiety increases the severity of the attack, so stay calm yourself and calm the child. Tell him or her that the doctor is on the way.

Sit the child up either in bed or in a chair and keep the room warm. If the child is taken to the doctor or to the hospital then he or she should be sat up, not laid down in the back of a car. It sometimes helps if the child leans forward onto a chair back or some pillows. This helps support the chest and enables the muscles to work at breathing more efficiently. Encourge the child to drink.

Drug treatment
Some drugs act by widening narrowed airways. These are called brochodilators and come in various forms including inhalers and liquids to take by mouth. Inhalers tend to work more efficiently and quickly, but young children are not always able to coordinate their breathing to use them correctly. Ask about the devices available to get round this such as inhalers which shoot out a measured dose of the drug into a plastic container. This retains the spray until the child breathes it in eliminating the need to breathe in at the exact moment that the drug is sprayed out.

Other drugs act by stabilizing the sensitive airways and preventing an asthma attack from ever starting. These need to be taken regularly as prescribed. This group of drugs will not, however, cure an acute attack once it has begun. Intal is the best known in this group and can only be taken by inhalation.

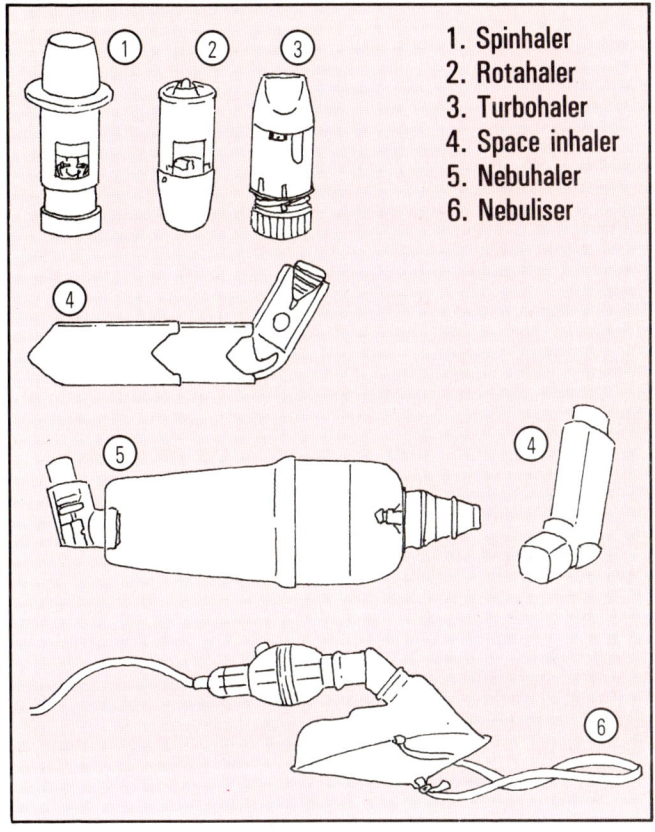

1. Spinhaler
2. Rotahaler
3. Turbohaler
4. Space inhaler
5. Nebuhaler
6. Nebuliser

There are a variety of methods of administering the correct doses of asthma treatments using the above devices.

The doctor may prescribe steroids. Do not be afraid of using these because they can be very helpful. They are usually given in inhaler form. Antibiotics may be necessary if the lungs are infected and the child has a temperature.

Physiotherapy
The child can be taught breathing exercises to help the symptoms during an attack.

Nebulizers
These machines are used to deliver drug treatment, (usually a bronchodilator — a drug to widen the airways) in a fine mist which can then be breathed in. They are very

effective if used correctly, and will get drugs to narrowed airways which inhalers have often failed to remedy. Few asthmatic children need to have one of their own at home.

Nebulizers are available in hospitals and many family doctors now carry them. They can be bought or borrowed and used at home by parents of sufferers without direct medical supervision. They are, however, only supplied to parents who understand their limitations, and usually after a specialist has assessed the problem.

It is possible to monitor the air flow in asthma with a simple meter. This can be used to detect when the nebulizer is needed and must be understood before a nebulizer is permitted in the house. The level of air flow at which the nebulizer needs to be used, **despite other regular treatment**, will be agreed with your doctor beforehand. The meter can then be used to monitor the effect of the nebulizer.

BEWARE of overrelying on nebulizers. Call the doctor if you nebulize your child once and breathing does not improve dramatically. Keep on with the child's other treatments while using the nebulizer.

Because nebulizers are so effective, many professionals fear that parents will go on using them with the child deteriorating dangerously. Ideally all asthmatics should have a peak flow meter to measure their performance every day. When they are deteriorating, they should increase their medication and seek advice if no improvement is made. Nebulizers are not the answer for everyone, some of the other gadgets are just as effective.

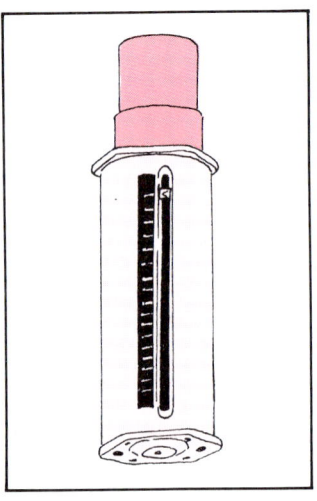

A nebulizer must be used in conjunction with a peak flow meter (left) which monitors the air flow and indicates when the nebulizer is needed.

Exercise

Exercise can help asthmatics and swimming is especially beneficial. Some exertion, however, particularly in cold weather can make things worse. Encourage asthmatic children not to think of themselves as invalids. If exercise does bring wheezing on then use inhalers before games.

Other triggers

Anxiety is often a factor in asthmatic attacks. Most doctors know wheezy children who get better once they know they are going to see the doctor. Children also start to wheeze because of worries about certain situations they find stressful. These can often be identified and put right.

Asthma can also be brought on as a reaction to an allergen like the house dust mite. Identify the problem and then work to avoid it.

Babies with asthma

Some young babies, under the age of about eighteen months, become wheezy after a viral chest cold. At one time these children were said to have a condition called wheezy bronchitis. More recently there has been a growing awareness amongst doctors that it is probably because these children are asthmatic. The correct diagnosis is important if the child is to be treated with the appropriate medicine.

The wheeziness is caused by the small air passages becoming inflamed and clogged with mucus. As well as the wheeze the child is feverish, breathes rapidly and looks unwell.

The doctor will usually need to see the child to confirm the diagnosis and see if antibiotics are needed to prevent complications. Quite often these children are so unwell that they need to go into hospital for a night or two.

Do not be alarmed by a diagnosis of asthma. It is merely a word which means wheeziness. Its importance lies in the fact that it makes parents and doctors see to it that your child gets proper treatment.

Treatment

The child may need antibiotics if he or she has a temperature. If asthma is diagnosed specific asthma treatments may be prescribed. Physiotherapy is sometimes helpful to bring up the plugs of white sputum. Until quite recently this was the mainstay of treatment as asthma wasn't always recognized for what it was.

Cough medicines are not helpful. At best they are useless and at worse they stop the child bringing up the plugs of sputum.

Remember that most children will grow out of wheezy attacks and will probably not suffer a life of chronic asthma.

Food intolerance

Some children appear to be intolerant or allergic to certain foodstuffs. There has been a lot of interest in food allergies recently and although they are far from understood the signs are that is it is much more common than previously suspected.

Many food allergies are obvious. The child who gets hives after eating strawberries is a clear example. A few cases of illnesses such as eczema, migraine and hyperactivity seem to benefit from changes in diet but unfortunately there is no easy way to relate symptoms to diet.

Problem foods
There are a great number of foods that may cause allergic reactions and it is impossible to list them all here. The more common ones are cow's milk, fruit, eggs, chocolate, cane sugar and various food colourings and preservatives contained in processed foods.

Diagnosis
Try to find a link between a particular food and a particular set of symptoms. Suspect a food allergy if there is a family history of allergy, or if the child suffers with other clear allergic problems, such as asthma.

Treatment
Identify the problem and avoid it. Do not put a child on a food exclusion diet without medical advice. If you exclude the wrong things, the child's growth could suffer.

Discuss the subject of food intolerance with your doctor. There are various drugs available and as this is a very specialized and advancing area of medicine, with your doctor's approval the child could well be referred to a specialist.

Headaches and migraine

Headaches are very common in childhood and the word migraine is a very loose term. A lot of headaches are described as migraine when they are not. There is quite a lot of overlap between tension headaches, which are common and migraine itself. A classic migraine headache is on one side of the head and is associated with sickness and temporary changes in vision. Children do suffer from migraine but not usually with the same symptoms as adults.

Abdominal migraine

The reason it is called this is because the major symptoms are nausea and tummy ache. This term is not a perfect one. Over the years the symptoms have had a variety of names which really just indicates how unclear the exact problem often is. The severity of the symptoms varies a lot and can be quite severe with fever and vomiting.

About half these children grow out of the attacks. A few go on to develop the typical adult pattern of symptoms indicating that migraine may in fact be the cause of a child getting repeated bouts of tummy ache for which no cause can be found. The symptoms often coincide with periods of stress such as going to school on a Monday morning. There is often a family history of migraine.

Treatment

You cannot alter the personality of your child but understanding the problem helps. The medical treatment of migraine-type headaches in childhood usually only involves a simple painkiller such as paracetamol. This drug is very effective. The doctor may need to prescribe a drug to ease any nausea and sickness.

Very rarely childhood headaches are due to something more serious. If your child's headache persists, go and see your family doctor.

Nettle rash (hives)

This allergic skin rash has a number of causes and looks like nettle stings. A chemical called histamine is released by the body into the skin and produces white lumpy wheals of various sizes on a reddened skin. The rash is very itchy and may go completely after an hour or so, or it can disappear, only to break out elsewhere on the body.

The cause may be obvious (if the child falls into a bed of stinging nettles) or it may be quite obscure. Foods such as shellfish and strawberries are often involved. Drugs such as penicillin can produce such a rash. Occasionally a child's skin reacts this way to insect bites.

Treatment
Put calamine lotion onto the wheals and leave it to dry without touching it. This may settle the reaction. The next thing to try is a warm bath with half a cup of baking soda (sodium bicarbonate).

In the long-term, do some detective work to find out what triggered off the rash. Aspirin, for example, is a common cause but often not suspected because it is a medicine! If you suspect a food such as shellfish, cut it out of the diet for a few weeks, then reintroduce it and see what happens.

Calling the doctor
Very occasionally this form of allergic reaction can be severe. The doctor needs to see the child quickly, particularly if the swelling is in or around the mouth. He or she may prescribe an antihistamine drug.

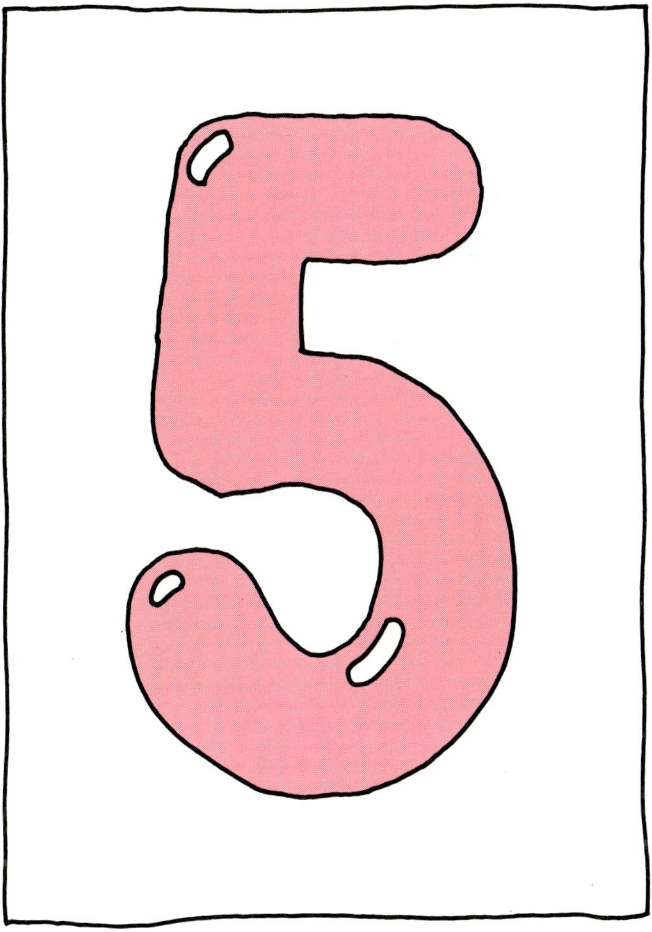

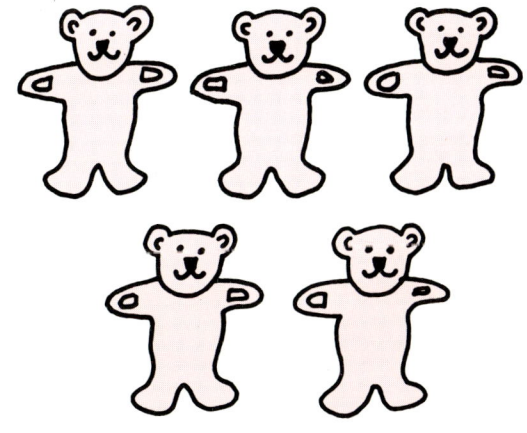

Ears and eyes

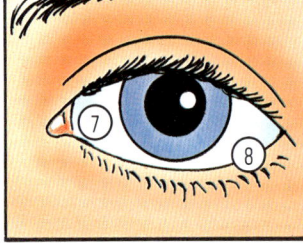

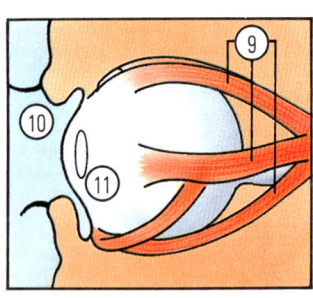

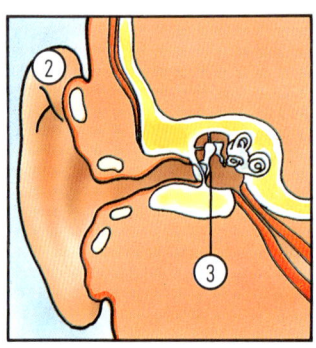

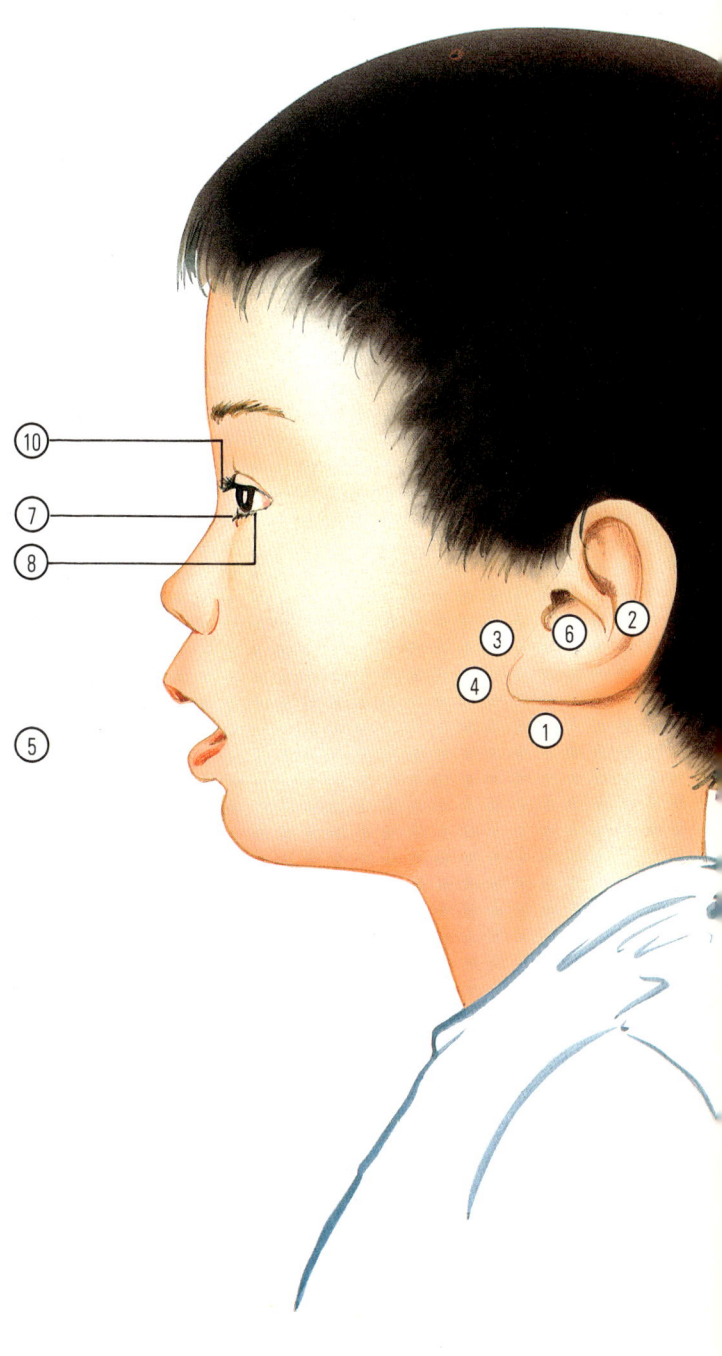

Ears and eyes

Ears

The ears are not just organs of hearing, they also have sensitive mechanisms deep inside them which maintain our balance.

The outer ear

Gristly flaps called pinnae stick out of each side of the head. They do not cause many health problems except that parents sometimes worry that they stick out too much and that the child is bat-eared. An older child may get teased at school. If you are really concerned, talk to your doctor about them. In a few cases a simple cosmetic operation is all that is necessary to correct the problem. This is not usually done until after a child is about six. Do not waste time and tape sticking the ears down or concern yourself that the way the pinna lies on the pillow at night will make the problem any better or worse.

The external ear canal is a tunnel from the pinna to the eardrum and is lined with cells which produce a soft, yellow wax which naturally moves up the canal to the outside clearing away dust and debris which may collect in the canal. The start of the canal is the hole down which a finger can be poked. Pushing things into the ear canal will impact the wax which builds up and hardens into dark orange masses further down in the canal.

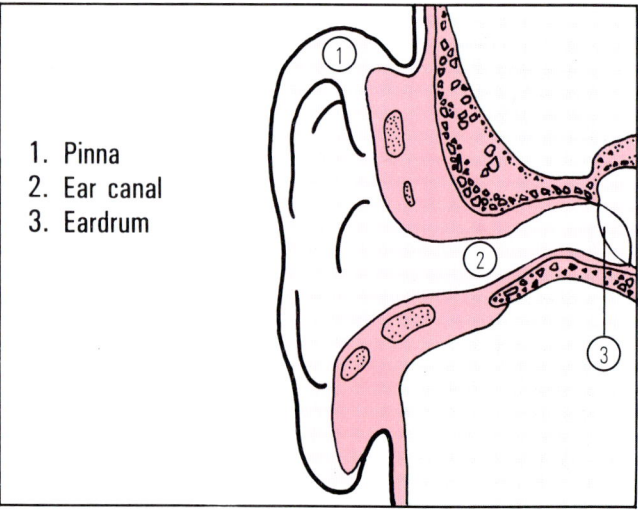

1. Pinna
2. Ear canal
3. Eardrum

Otitis externa

The ear canal is the passage the doctor looks down to see the eardrum. If this canal gets inflamed the condition is called otitis externa. The pain and problem is external to the eardrum and it hurts to move the pinna.

This inflammation is quite common in children. The common cause of this is cleaning ears out with a cotton bud or fingers. Ears only need washing, not cleaning out. Wax is good and there for a purpose. Another cause is a foreign body, such as a bead or pea, which has been poked into the ear canal or swimming, especially in chlorinated water. If you suspect otitis externa, your child needs to be taken to the doctor (see also eczema, page 120).

Treatment is to remove any cause and then treat with antibiotics either by mouth or in drops. The drops may also contain some form of anti-inflammatory drug.

Sometimes, instead of a general inflammation in the canal there is a localized problem such as a boil and it is quite common not to find the cause of this with any certainty.

Foreign bodies

Young children (sometimes with a little help from their friends) occasionally poke things into the ear. The most usual objects are beads and pieces of paper. These may be quite difficult to get out if you do not have both experience and the right instruments. Beads, for example, are round and smooth and tend to get pushed towards the eardrum. This can be painful and makes the whole incident worse.

My advice is that unless the child keeps still and the object can be easily seen and grabbed without fuss using tweezers, get expert help. From my experience of removing things from children's ears, this combination is rare if the bead is well and truly impacted. In fact, I cannot recall a young child who sat quietly when approached to have something removed from the ear!

Sometimes things are found in the ear on routine examination. I know of one man who was deaf in one ear nearly all his life. At the age of seventy six, a rolled up bus ticket shot out of the ear when his wife slapped him on the back. It was dated 1927. It had been partially blocking his ear for 60 years. Hopefully if your child does this it will be detected a bit sooner.

You can help prevent children poking around in their ears by not doing it yourself. It is not necessary to probe inside children's ears with cotton buds or rolled corners of towels at bath time. Water and wax run out on their own given time. Wax is a natural part of the body. Simply wipe it away as it reaches the outer ear.

Something may be in the ear if:

- The child tells you
- The ear is painful
- Hearing is reduced

The middle ear is an air-filled chamber housed in the bones of the skull. The Eustachian tube (1) opens out at the back of the throat. Three tiny auditory ossicles (2) transmit vibrations from the eardrum (3) to the inner ear (4) where sound is registered in the coiled cochlea (5). The semi-circular canals (6) control balance.

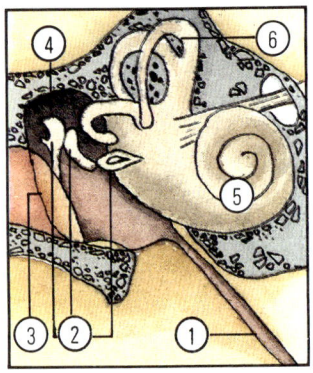

The middle ear

The eardrum is a circular clear window between the external ear canal and the cave-like middle ear. A healthy drum looks and acts exactly like the skin of a real drum. It is a very sensitive membrane and changes in air pressure on either side of it can alone produce the discomfort and popping many people experience when going up in an aeroplane. If it is stretched by infection or touched by anything that has been pushed down the ear canal then the pain is dreadful.

The middle ear is an air-filled chamber on the other side of the eardrum. Three tiny bones called the auditory ossicles stretch from the eardrum on one side of the chamber to a smaller drum which connects with the auditory nerve of the brain. These tiny bones conduct vibrations of sound across the middle ear to the auditory nerve and thus to the brain where the vibrations are translated into sound. The middle ear also has a tiny tube which runs down to the back of the throat. This is called the Eustachian tube.

Otitis media

This is an infection of the middle ear and the commonest cause of earache. Germs can spread from the throat into the middle ear up the Eustachian tube. This usually happens after one of the head colds that are so common in young children. The germs find it relatively easy to track up the Eustachian tube because in children under about six years of age the tube is short and wide. Also babies spend more time lying down and gravity helps the germs on their way.

To make matters worse there may be enlarged adenoids at the outlet of the tube into the throat. This can hold up drainage from the chamber of the middle ear, and fluids and secretion which stagnate can very quickly get infected.

Symptoms

Otitis media in young children can be difficult to detect. Older children usually complain of pain. Although the most common symptom is earache, a small baby cannot tell you what the problem is.

The only sign may be that the child is obviously ill, running a high fever and in pain. In fact, a doctor usually checks the ears of children who are feverish and unwell for no apparent cause.

Sometimes otitis media is almost symptomless, but the child just seems a little deaf. If you suspect this, get the doctor to check.

Treatment

Initially paracetamol and a decongestant like Sudafed may be all that is needed to relieve the child's symptoms while you wait for a suitable time to see the doctor.

If the condition worsens the mainstay of treatment prescribed by the doctor is an antibiotic by mouth. (Ear drops of course are of no use since the eardrum separates the middle ear from the outside world.) Sometimes nose drops are used as well to help the middle ear drain down the Eustachian tube. For the same reason a decongestant taken by mouth may be prescribed.

This kind of treatment will nearly always settle a bout of this form of ear infection as long as the whole course of treatment is completed. If, however, the child gets repeated attacks which start to affect hearing and general health, then your doctor is likely to consider asking an ear nose and throat specialist to advise. At this stage some kind of operation may be considered.

Runny ear

If anything runs out of the ear consult the doctor. The cause may simply be wax, but if an infection builds up in the middle ear and does not get treatment the eardrum may burst allowing a mixture of pus and blood to escape which you may see as a discharge on the child's pillow. Once the infection is treated a perforated eardrum usually heals quickly.

Glue ear

This looks like it sounds. The middle ear and Eustachian tube fill up with sticky mucus which affects hearing. It is a painless condition best imagined as a big bass drum that has had treacle poured into it. Imagine the poor quality of sound you would get when you tried to beat it. The same bad transmission happens in the middle ear. Noise from the outside world is muffled in its journey to the brain. Glue ear is an important cause of poor speech development in children. They do not hear the sounds properly and they repeat them as they hear them.

The condition seems to be becoming increasingly common, possibly because of the increased use (and misuse) of antibiotics. Our parents had to contend with serious infections and abscesses of the middle ear (penicillin was not available until the 1940s). These are uncommon now and the serious forms are rare because antibiotics are available to kill the bacteria that cause the problem. The sticky mucus of glue ear is not an infective problem, however, and one reason why it may be more common is that children are not made to finish a course of antibiotics. Fluid builds up in the middle ear as a result of chronic infection and cannot drain away down a blocked Eustachian tube.

Symptoms
Because there is often no pain the first thing you are likely to notice about your child is that his or her hearing is less than perfect. A child has the television on too loud, or turns one ear (the good one) towards a sound. Children rarely pretend to be deaf. If your child appears not to hear, ask your doctor to check.

Try calling your child quietly from behind. If he or she fails to turn round, or seems uncertain where the sound is coming from, the problem needs further investigation. Try

A grommet is placed through the eardrum to keep a channel open between the outer and middle ear.

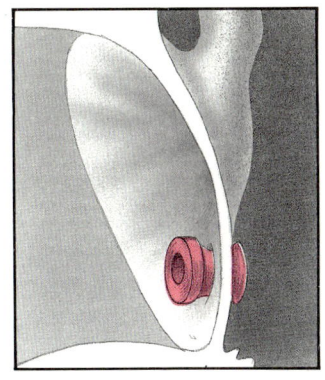

this test when one of your child's friends is in the house so that you can compare two children of the same age, assuming that the friend has not got hearing problems as well!

Hearing problems are very common around the age children start school. (About 20 in every 1000 are likely to be affected.) One vital reason to find these children and treat them is that their schooling may suffer if no one realizes that they cannot hear lessons properly.

Treatment

Go and see the doctor who can look at the eardrum and see if it looks clear. Also he or she can test your child's hearing. For a first attack medicines (although not necessarily antibiotics) can be taken by mouth to dry out the ear.

If this does not sort the problem out the doctor will consider asking an ear, nose and throat specialist for an opinion and an operation may be done to insert small tubes called grommets into the eardrum.

Grommets are tiny, short tubes. Their role is to keep the pressure equal on either side of the eardrum by maintaining a hole. Left to itself the eardrum, being made of skin, quickly heals up. The grommets either fall out on their own or are taken out by the specialist leaving the small hole in the drum to heal up. Hearing should then return to normal.

During the operation any underlying problem like unhealthy tonsils and adenoids may be dealt with under the same general anaesthetic. If both ears are affected then the child will have grommets in both ears.

After this simple operation it is important to keep the ears dry, so take the advice of the specialist about swimming and the need to wear ear plugs in the pool and in the bath at home. Some people recommend using Blutac.

Causes of earache

● **Otitis externa**
(a) inflammation down ear canal
(b) boil in ear canal
(c) foreign body down ear canal

● **Otitis media**
Eustachian tube gets blocked during a cold and with no outlet to keep pressure equal, the eardrum gets sucked in. Pus and infection form in the middle ear cavity.

● **Mumps**
The parotid gland swells and is very close to the ear.

● **Toothache**
Pain from a tooth can seem to come from the ear. The side of the face is quite a difficult area of the body to pinpoint exact areas of pain — there are so many tissues close together with nerves in close contact.

● **Foreign body**
If wax or anything else (such as a bead) is poked down to touch the sensitive drum.

Call the doctor if:

● It hurts to move the child's pinna.
● You suspect a foreign body is in the ear.
● The child is running a high fever and complaining of painful ears.
● After a head cold the child seems a little deaf or the ears are causing pain.
● Anything runs out of the ear.
● If you notice any behaviour which might suggest deafness.
● There is pain when you tap the hard round bump just behind the pinna (mastoid bone).

Assessing hearing

Good hearing is essential for proper development. Children learn to speak from the things they hear and they learn at school by listening. The term deaf mute comes from the days when ear disease was more common and deafness very often went hand in hand with delayed speech.

Unfortunately, testing a child's hearing is not as easy as taking a temperature with a thermometer. You need to know the signs of poor hearing, and these tend to vary with age.

Under four months
It is very hard to test hearing with any accuracy. Your child should respond in some way to a voice or familiar noise and will gurgle back when spoken to.

Four to twelve months
Babies in this age group should be making noises of their own more and more. A few with a hearing problem will be quiet because they are not aware of sounds around them. They will not join in with their parents in the charming smiling, gurgling way that normal babies do.

By the time a normal baby is coming up to a year old, loud sounds may be deliberately ignored. The baby is beginning to realize that it is not necessary to react to every sound. Paradoxically, it is about this time a child with poor hearing may start reacting to loud noises.

One to two years
A child starts to speak words and build short sentences during the second year of life. The timing of this is much more variable than many parents expect, as are other milestones such as rolling over, standing and walking. If, however, you feel that your child is lagging behind, talk to the doctor or health visitor.

End of first year at school
At the risk of being boring it has to be repeated yet again that poor hearing handicaps a child's development. The child cannot learn because he or she cannot hear. Teachers may become concerned that all is not well. Talk to your doctor or health visitor if you have any anxieties and a hearing test can be arranged.

Preventing deafness

● Get vaccinated against German measles before getting pregnant (see pages 156-157). This is an easy way to eliminate one of the common causes of deafness from birth.

● Get ear infections cleared up quickly and fully. See the child finishes courses of antibiotics.

● Do not poke things down the ear even in an attempt to clean it.

● Loud noise damages hearing and it will not return. Older children should not be allowed to abuse such things as personal stereo headphones.

● Get a child's ears checked if you suspect any degree of deafness.

● Older children should be warned of the dangers of unreasonably loud music.

Eyes

The conjunctiva is a delicate membrane that lines the inside of the eyelids and covers the exposed front of the eyeball. If it becomes inflamed the eyes look bloodshot. The condition is called conjunctivitis and happens for a number of reasons. These can be divided into two groups, those caused by infections and those which are not! It is worth knowing the difference, because it helps in prevention and cure.

Infective conjunctivitis

This is caused by a bacteria or a virus. One or both eyes may be affected. Typically the eye is most sticky in the morning, when it may be almost stuck closed. This form of eye inflammation is often called pink eye.

Conjunctivitis is often a complication of the common cold when the tear ducts, which drain tears from the eyes to the nose, get blocked so that dust which lands on the eye cannot be washed away.

The conjunctivitis may exist on its own, or the child may be ill with something else. For example, conjunctivitis is a very common accompaniment to measles. Pink eye is easily spread around so the following rules about washing hands, touching the eyes, and using medicine correctly are important.

The conjunctiva is a thin protective membrane which lines the inside of the eyelids and the front of the eyeball itself.

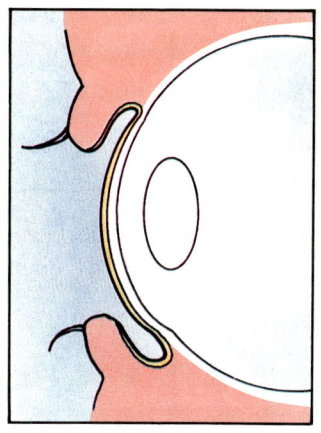

Home nursing

Discourage the child from rubbing the eyes. This makes the symptoms worse, and it may spread the infection. Without making too much of a fuss see that the child uses a separate towel and flannel while the eyes are infected.

Bathe any discharge away with cotton wool dipped in boiled water that has cooled. Start on the inside and work outwards and throw away the cotton wool to avoid spreading the problem.

Light may make the symptoms worse, so draw the curtains and avoid bright lights. The child may be willing to wear dark glasses as a temporary measure.

Treatment

If you think the eye has this type of infection, get medical help as antibiotics are probably needed. The antibiotics will probably be given either as drops or ointment.

Use the medicine exactly as the doctor has said, so be certain when you leave the surgery that you know how long to put it in, how many times a day, and if it is to go into only one or both eyes.

Do not share the medicine around if any of the other children go down with same infection. They will need their own medicine.

Throw away ointment or drops once the course has finished. Do not store a half-used tube for possible future problems because these medicines can get germs into them which makes the problem worse the next time you use them. Eye medicines seldom contain preservatives because these would irritate the sensitive eye.

Non-infective conjunctivitis

This is usually the result of an allergy or of something going into the eye. The eyes can become allergic to all sorts of things. The most common causes in children are probably those linked with hay fever. In the summer the pollens that can produce the classic hay-fever symptoms also cause red itchy eyes. The child may have other symptoms as well such as a runny nose and an allergic cough. (See Chapter 4, pages 42-56).

There are, however, many things that can cause an allergic conjunctivitis and in the less obvious cases it is something to consider carefully. It is a mistake to instantly assume that an itchy or gritty red eye is the result of an infection and needs antibiotics.

Some of the advice given for infective conjunctivitis will be helpful in these cases. So wipe away any discharge, and protect the eye with a pad or dark glasses. Check for a foreign body although many foreign bodies are too small to see unless the doctor stains the surface of the eye.

Work out what has caused the problem. It may be possible to avoid it.

Treatment
There are a number of treatments available to the doctor to treat allergic conjuntivitis and they usually come in the form of drops.

There are drops available which prevent the symptoms. These actually lock the stable door before the horse bolts! However, because they are actually preventative they take time to work and need perseverance. They do not provide the instant cure many people expect from modern medicine and sometimes are abandoned too quickly. If there are other allergic symptoms you may be prescribed one of the antihistamines. These are taken by mouth and have the advantage that they will act against all the symptoms of allergy. (So a child with a runny nose, itchy eyes and a tight wheezy chest does not have to leave the surgery with a prescription for three different medicines!)

There are two fairly new antihistamines which do not make patients sleepy. They are astemizole (Hismanal) and terfenadine (Triludan). Both are available without a prescription, but are not recommended in children under six. It is vital that the instructions are followed. Hismanal must be taken on an empty stomach or it may not work. Take it for several days before it exerts its full effect.

Foreign body in the eye

Children do not poke things into their eyes as they do into their ear and up their nose. If something goes in and stays in, it is likely to be a piece of grit, a fly, or perhaps dust or corn from a summer field. Only very occasionally is it metal or glass.

The eye is red, sore and watering; sometimes the eyesight is reduced. It may be possible to see the cause of the trouble. If the grit is under the upper lid the patient will tell you where it hurts. You cannot see something stuck under the upper lid without lifting the lid up and looking at the undersurface.

Important!

Never try to remove a foreign body from the coloured part of the eye. Do not try to dig anything out that is embedded in the eye.

Treatment

It is important not to rub the eye and make things worse. If the eye is watering it is helpful and you can encourage the eye to do this by rubbing the good eye. If you can see the foreign body, then it may be possible to gently lift it off. For example, if there is a fly on the lower part of the conjunctiva (the delicate membrane that lines the inside of the eyelids and covers the exposed part of the eyeball), this can usually be lifted off with the corner of a handkerchief or a cotton wool bud. If you've encouraged the child to blink the tears may wash something like this from the surface of the eye down into this position or pull the upper lid down over the lower one so that the lower eyelashes can pull out anything under the upper lid.

If the actual tears do not wash out the eye then you can use tap water. If you try to pour the fluid directly into the eye, the child will blink, but if you gently run warm water onto the forehead before you lower the jug and allow it to run into the eye, the child should be able to keep the eye open.

If the trouble is under the upper lid the child will probably tell you that this is where the scratching feeling is coming from. It is possible with a little bit of practice to turn this upper lid inside out but it isn't always an easy thing to do without some medical training. Even then it's

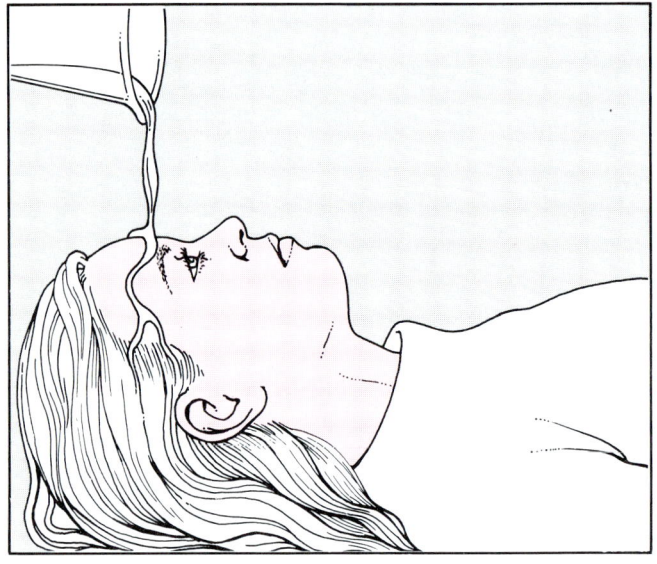

To irrigate a child's eye begin running warm water gently over the forehead then move the flow onto the eye. This should help the child to keep the eye open.

not easy. If you can't manage it, try looking under the lid by pulling the skin above the upper eyelid up. If there is trouble here and you can't clear it by irrigating with water, then you will need to get help.

After something has been in the eye and come out either of its own accord or because you have taken it out, the child may still feel that there is something there. This is because the surface of the eye has been scratched, but this unpleasant sensation will soon settle down.

Stye

A stye is a small pus-filled boil at the base of an eyelash. The eyelid is painful and begins to swell. The stye usually comes to a head and bursts on its own after four or five days.

Treatment
Styes are not usually serious and you can probably treat them without calling the doctor.

Encourage the child to leave the eye alone. Pulling an eyelid will make the pain worse. In fact doing this may have started the stye of in the first place. The eye can be protected from its owner's fingers with a clean eye pad.

The stye will probably burst of its own accord. As it comes to a head encourage this by bathing the area carefully with cotton wool dipped in warm water. If the abscess bursts wipe the pus away.

Take the child to the doctor if the problem keeps coming back, or if the stye appears not to settle within a week. Remember the best treatment for any abscess like this is for it to drain away. Antibiotics in fact are usually not necessary and may drag the problem out by delaying the discharge of the pus.

Squints

Before the age of three to six months, a baby's eyes may not always work together in a perfectly coordinated way. To some degree they may act independently so the baby can appear to have a small squint from time to time but not at all times. Any obvious or constant squint is abnormal even at this young age and it can be difficult to tell the difference. If you do suspect that the eyes are not working together properly and that there is a squint present, it is better to see your doctor, so that you can be sure whether the appearance you have noticed is acceptable or not.

By the age of six months, the two eyes will be working together so that each eye looks as though it is linked to the other and they move exactly together in whatever direction they are directed. It is important to do something about any abnormality because the treatment of a squint is much more effective if it is undertaken quickly at a young age. When an eye starts to squint, the baby's brain prevents the confusion of double vision because it is able to ignore one of the two separate pictures that it is receiving. This suppression of the vision from the squinting eye can be very difficult to reverse if it goes untreated for long enough, and we arc talking about months rather than weeks. If it is not treated before the age of three or four years at the latest, then this eye can have permanently lazy vision.

The most common cause of squint developing in a child is that there is far- or nearsightedness present and as this is usually greater in one eye, then this is the eye that tends to squint. Glasses therefore not only help the child to control

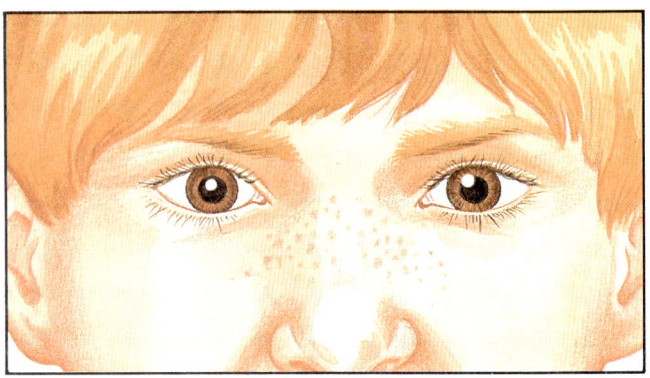

Highlights should fall in exactly the same place on the pupil of both eyes whatever direction the child looks. If they don't there may be a squint so get advice.

the squint, but also improve the vision. Extra treatment such as exercises and sometimes even an operation may be needed to treat a squint.

Another common cause for a squint developing is that the muscles that move the eyes are not properly balanced. A squint can also appear because one eye has some problem inside it which prevents it seeing normally. All these reasons make it important for you to consult your family doctor if you think that your child does have a squint.

Recognizing a squint

The squint may be obvious, or other people may tell you. Get the child to look at a toy or finger and move this around. The squint may only be obvious when the eyes look in a certain direction.

It is not always easy to decide on this and I speak from personal experience. Both my children started squinting at the age of about one and we found they were farsighted. So get medical advice.

Some children only appear to squint because of the shape of the face. The eyeball does not sit symmetrically in its socket. Your child will be checked at different stages of development but if you suspect a squint go to the doctor straight away. The earlier treatment begins the better. The longer you wait the greater the danger of permanent loss of eyesight.

Recognizing a child needs glasses
- The child may start to squint (like my children). This is usually much earlier than the age when a child will actually be able to tell you they cannot see.
- Older children will screw their eyes up and peer at the blackboard or television. They may or may not actually tell you. Often they will not because they do not know what perfect vision is like.
- Get the child's eyes checked yearly if there is any question about the way the eyes are working.

Common questions

Will my child always have to wear glasses?
Not necessarily. Eyes change a great deal up to puberty. This is particularly so in farsighted eyes when the degree of farsightedness can reduce markedly. The changes that take place, however, are not likely to mean that a very longsighted child can go without some form of glasses. Nearsightedness may increase as the child gets older and is uncommon before the age of five or six.

Can the child go over to contact lenses at some stage?
Yes, but it is only very occasionally that young children need contact lenses. In general, they are not a good idea because a young child cannot manage them easily.

From experience of our own children, it is easy for the child to get upset about wearing glasses at first, but it is important to encourage a child to keep them on. My advice (unless you are incredibly rich) is not to spend a fortune on the frames because the lenses are the important part. Keep a spare pair in case of accidents.

However, as a child gets older he or she may prefer contact lenses which are cosmetically more pleasing. Incidentally, they are easier to tolerate in nearsightedness than farsightedness because of the shape of the lens.

Why does my child see the orthoptist?
The orthoptist works together with the specialist (opthalmologist) as part of a team. The orthoptist does two basic things when seeing your child. She measures the degree of squint and can monitor the response of the eye to glasses or any operations that are carried out.

The second thing she is concerned with is measuring vision. This is a very skilled procedure in a child too young to read an eye chart.

What does the eye specialist or opthalmologist do?
The specialist tends to be the coordinator of the orthoptist/specialist team. Most of the treatment is based on information from the orthoptist. The orthoptist does the measuring and recording, the ophthalmologist does the operating. He or she may also prescribe glasses as does the optician.

Surgery may be necessary to adjust one of the eye muscles. Glasses can compensate for far or nearsightedness, and if one eye is lazy then exercises may be recommended. Patching the good eye is a form of exercise because it forces the child to use the muscles of the lazy eye.

What does a farsighted and nearsighted child actually see?
A farsighted child usually sees a fairly normal world. The eyes are very good at accommodating for farsightedness, but if one eye finds this too much of an effort, then this is when a squint can develop.

A nearsighted child has trouble seeing things like the blackboard and television. It actually depends on how nearsighted he or she is, but things beyond about arm's length tend to be blurred.

Does a squint always mean a child is far or nearsighted?
No. Sometimes a squint develops because the muscles that move the eyeball have not learnt to move together. A squint can therefore develop in a normally sighted eye.

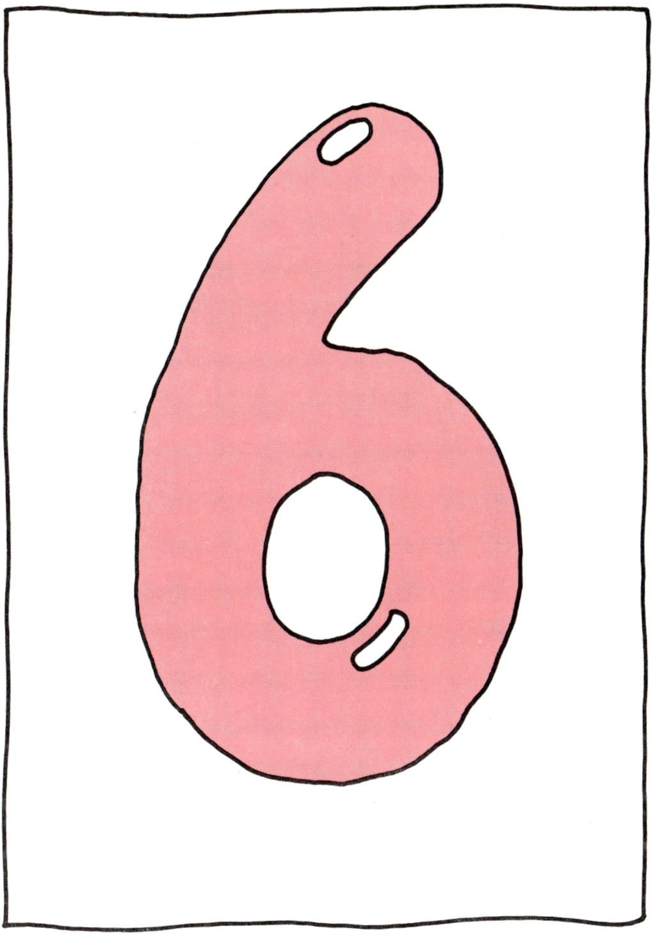

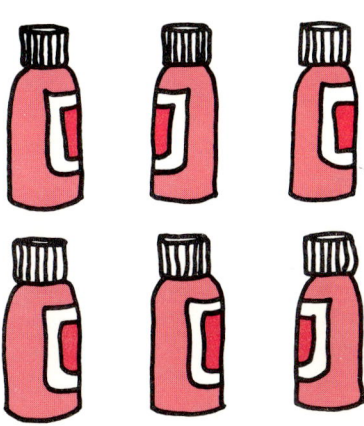

Tummy troubles

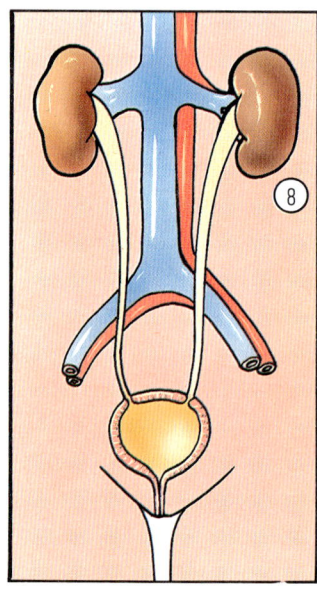

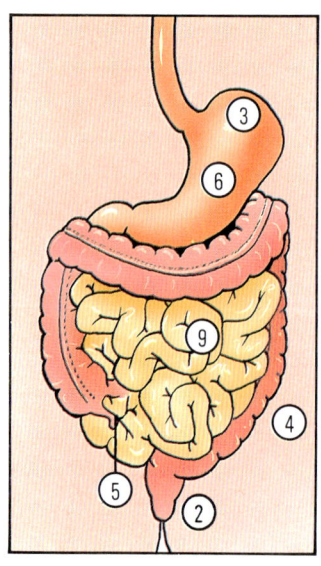

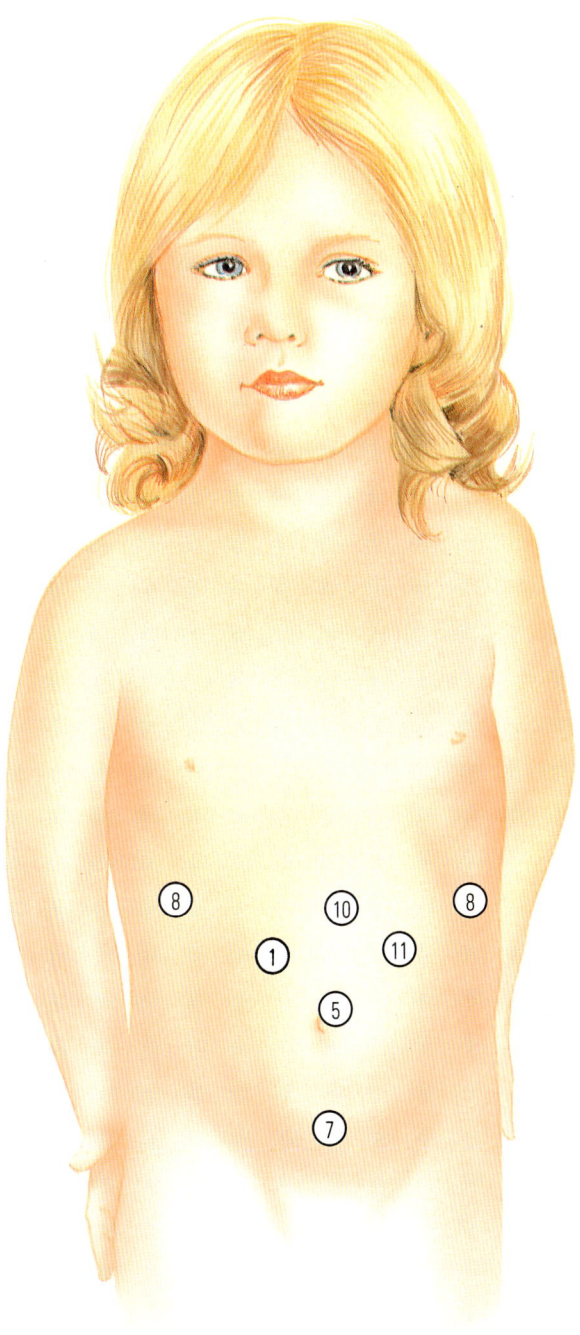

Tummy troubles

Tummy ache

More than half of the bouts of tummy ache that your child suffers will go away without any cause ever being found. These bouts can be painful and distressing, but armed with the knowledge that the pain is not a sign of a serious condition such as appendicitis or a twisted bowel, you can offer the support and comfort a child needs.

Signs and symptoms

It is helpful to know exactly what you are talking about when you describe abdominal problems because sometimes the terms are misused and misunderstood. Each of the following symptoms is discussed in full further on in this chapter.

Colic is pain in the abdomen which comes in waves. It can be quite severe.

Constipation is a delay in emptying the bowels which causes the stools to become hard and dry and makes them difficult to pass.

Vomiting occurs when muscle contractions throw the contents of the stomach out of the mouth. Do not confuse this with posseting in young babies which is the regurgitation of small amounts of milk after a feed.

Diarrhoea means the frequent passing of watery stools. It may be accompanied by waves of colic.

Colic

A number of internal organs have a muscle supply which we can't consciously control. Thus the intestines are able to squeeze food along without the owner of the body having to think about it. It is probably spasm of these muscles which causes the pain. In children, almost all colic is painful but unimportant. Worry only if the pain lasts for a couple of hours. There are a number of serious causes of intestinal colic, ranging from inflammation of the appendix, to obstruction of the bowel and food poisoning.

Intestinal colic is common in people of all age groups from babies to the very old. It can be very painful, but is usually harmless. In babies it is called three-month colic because this is age group that seems to be most distressed by it. It is a rather vague term for a common condition which affects a number of healthy babies.

Typically a baby, usually under the age of four months, draws up the legs, goes red in the face and screams in bouts, usually at a particular time of the day. This is generally attributed to intestinal colic, and it may well be the cause in some cases. However alarming it appears, it is worth saying that babies naturally draw their legs up like this when they cry. It does not necessarily mean that their tummy hurts. The sorts of colic which cause great pain in adults, for example renal colic from a stone in the kidney or biliary colic from a stone near the gall bladder, are not common childhood illnesses.

Having established that nothing is seriously amiss, parents are still left with the problem of handling what can become a very stressful situation. There is no instant certain cure, the phase will pass, but until it does:

1. Discuss the problem, not just with your doctor or health visitor, but also with your partner and other adults. This passing phase can cause a lot of stress and anxiety which simply makes things worse. The baby may well respond positively to a happier, less fraught atmosphere. In some cases your doctor may prescribe medicine.

2. With the help of your partner, try various ways of pacifying the child without letting the screaming get to you. (This is easier said than done.) Cuddle the baby, provide a feed or nappy change, carry him or her around in your arms or in the pram. Take the baby for a drive in the car or let him or her look over your shoulder as you pace about. You may find something which settles your baby.

Constipation

Most parents think they know what is meant by constipation, but often they don't and their misapprehensions can be passed onto the children. Unfortunately this will produce another generation of adults who are obsessed with bowels and bowel action. Children vary in their need to have their bowels open, some going twice a day, others once every three to four days. The consistency of the stool is much more important than the time between bowel actions.

Causes

By far and away the commonest cause of chronic constipation is worry about the bowels transmitted from over-anxious parents. Chronic constipation should not need any treatment because it should not be allowed to develop in the first place.

A child may have a bowel motion less frequently when he or she is ill with one of the minor childhood illnesses. The child is drinking less and may be sweating excessively and the body compensates for this by taking fluid from the stools. This type of constipation will settle by itself when the child gets back into a natural rhythm again.

General advice

Do not allow the child to become obsessed with bowel actions. He or she will develop a satisfactory routine without interference from an adult. It may be after breakfast because the first meal of the day produces action at the other end. However, not everybody lives life in exactly the same way, so let the child choose the best time. If you are concerned, do not allow the child to feel this. Just tactfully keep an eye, ear or nose open.

Don't make a very young child sit for ages on a potty if he or she is expected to perform a miracle and cannot. Allow older children privacy and time to go to the toilet.

Give your children the right kind of healthy high fibre diet. Diet is a very important factor and conditions such as constipation, appendicitis, cancer of the bowel, varicose veins, anal fissures and piles are Western diseases which are virtually unknown in developing countries where the diet is high in fibre.

Constipation is very rare amongst breast-fed babies because mother's milk is such a good food. It is more common when babies are bottle fed and also is seen when babies go over to solid foods. Again this can be avoided by eating the right diet of vegetables and fresh fruit.

Give your children the right kind of healthy high fibre diet. High fibre vegetables and fruit are natural bulking agents. Diet is a very important factor and conditions such as constipation, appendicitis, cancer of the bowel, varicose veins, anal fissures and piles are Western diseases which are virtually unknown in developing countries where the diet is high in fibre.

It should hardly ever be necessary for parents to use chemical laxatives without having consulted the doctor.

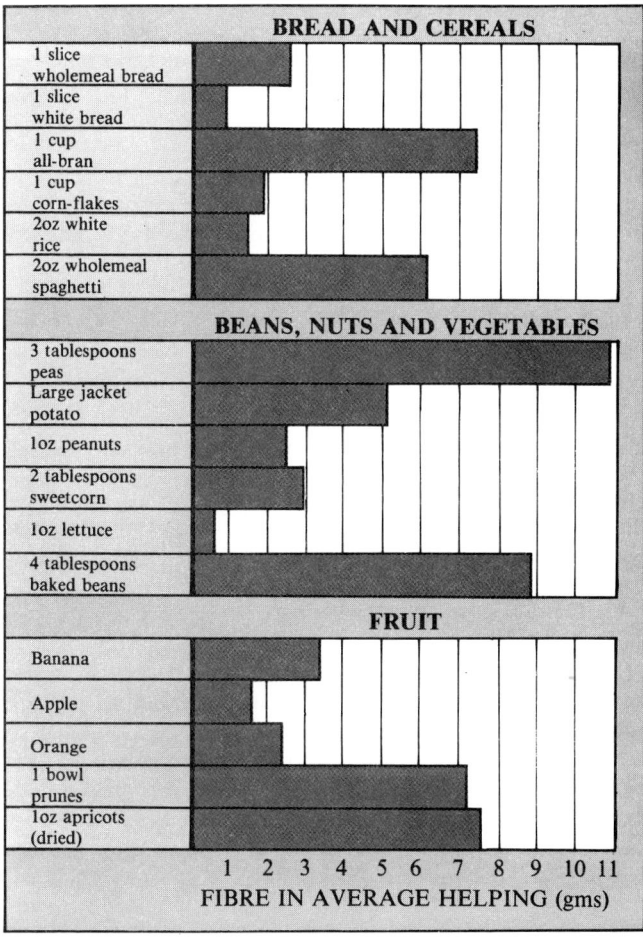

BREAD AND CEREALS

	1	2	3	4	5	6	7	8	9	10	11
1 slice wholemeal bread											
1 slice white bread											
1 cup all-bran											
1 cup corn-flakes											
2oz white rice											
2oz wholemeal spaghetti											

BEANS, NUTS AND VEGETABLES

3 tablespoons peas											
Large jacket potato											
1oz peanuts											
2 tablespoons sweetcorn											
1oz lettuce											
4 tablespoons baked beans											

FRUIT

Banana											
Apple											
Orange											
1 bowl prunes											
1oz apricots (dried)											

FIBRE IN AVERAGE HELPING (gms)

The doctor may use them in certain cases, but if constipation really does exist and is a problem it can usually be put right naturally without any fuss or drugs.

Call the doctor if:
- The child has abdominal pain. Constipation may cause this but so can other things, such as appendicitis.
- The child passes any blood. A hard motion can tear the anal margin and cause bleeding.
- Your home remedies, or more importantly your lack of home concern and interference, have not worked. There are a very few rare causes of constipation and the doctor can make sure that your child is basically healthy.

Vomiting

Although vomiting is always distressing, it can be caused by a number of conditions, some of which are not serious.

Overeating

Children who go to a party and eat and drink as much as possible, get excited and then come home and are sick are known to us all. Some children seem to be more sensitive than others.

Emotional

Some children vomit when they get upset. This can sometimes be interwoven with battles with parents over food and eating. These sorts of battles are best avoided because they give everybody indigestion.

Infection

Children very often vomit at the start of an infection such as tonsillitis, inflammation in the ear, or a kidney infection.

Travel sickness

If the child is going to suffer with this, it usually begins after the age of six months and a child nearly always grows out of it.

Reading in the car seems to make things worse, and watching the road often makes it better. The best way to prevent travel sickness, however, is to give the child one of the proprietary medicines available. Some preparations work better in some children than others, so its worth trying a variety until you find the one that suits your child the best.

Vomiting may be a symptom of a more serious illness. The following conditions are discussed in full later in the chapter.
- Appendicitis
- Gastroenteritis and food poisoning
- Blockage of the intestine
- Meningitis (see page 36)
- Migraine (see page 71)

Diarrhoea

Excessive fluid loss is the chief danger of diarrhoea.

Antisocial as it is, it very often doesn't do children any harm, unless fluid loss causes them to dry out. It is often accompanied by vomiting, whatever the cause.

The colour of what is passed may change if the intestinal contents hurry through a child quickly. In particular the stools may be an alarming bright green. This is because of green bile, which normally would have time to change to a more familiar brown colour, and is not a serious sign in itself nor is it an indication that a baby is starving.

Antibiotics may kill the cleansing bacteria which inhabit the bowel. This may cause temporary diarrhoea. Anxiety can also cause a temporary bout of diarrhoea because adrenaline speeds up the passage of food.

Diarrhoea may be a symptom of a more serious illness. The following conditions are discussed in full later in the chapter.
● Gastroenteritis and food poisoning
● Appendicitis

What to do
Call the doctor if you are not certain of the cause or if you know it is going to need treatment. It is impossible to give strict guidelines but if a child is not improving after 24 hours then you should get medical help. This does not mean, however, that the doctor should not be contacted before if you are worried about the child.

The mainstay of treatment is safe and simple and is saving millions of children all over the world. The child needs to take fluids by mouth. Breast milk is fine, if the child is still being fed in this way.

In older children the traditional method was to give them cool, boiled water in small sips. This will still do in an emergency, but there are now a number of products which come in different flavours and can be made up into a mixture. They usually come in powder form in sachets and are a mixture of glucose and salts. Follow the instructions on these and experiment to see which one your child likes. Replacing the fluids like this will keep most children healthy until the diarrhoea settles. The sachets are available without prescription, and are well worth having in the house ready for such emergencies. If a child is not able to tolerate fluids by mouth (which is unusual with these new products) then the child will have to go into hospital to have fluids into a vein until symptoms settle.

Do not worry about the child not eating while this is going on. Fluids, not food, are the vital thing.

Babies are much more vulnerable to fluid loss from diarrhoea than older children.

Dehydration

This is the big danger with diarrhoea and vomiting.

Signs and symptoms
The child who has lost a lot of fluid through diarrhoea and vomiting is drowsy and unwell. The lips and tongue may look dry, and the sign that doctors look for is a loss in the normal elasticity in the skin. If you gently pinch normal skin over an area like the chest, it will spring straight back into shape in a healthy child. In the dehydrated child, it is much less elastic and looks like old skin. As well as this the child's eyes may be sunken. Be on the look out for it if a child is continuing to loose fluid by vomiting and diarrhoea.

This chart shows the recommended daily fluid intake for children during illness. It can be given in any form the child finds palatable, but there are rehydration powders on the market which contain glucose and salts as well.

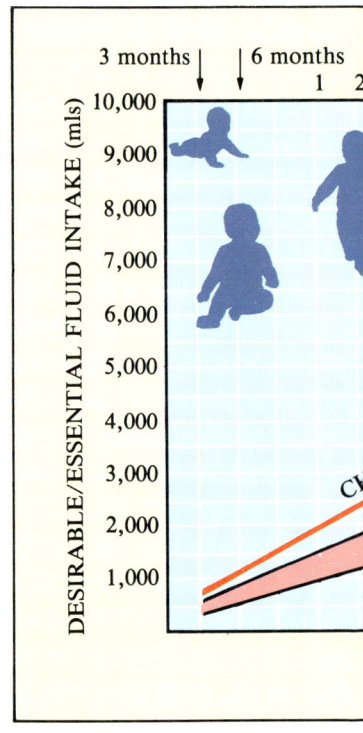

Gastroenteritis

Gastroenteritis is an inflammation of the stomach and small intestine which is usually caused by a virus. There are other germs and toxins which cause it. Breast feeding and a good standard of hygiene make it less common.

Signs and symptoms
Diarrhoea is the main symptom. The stools are green and watery and smell very unpleasant. The child can actually be quite well if it's a mild case but more severely affected children look ill, may have a fever, may vomit and may show signs of dehydration.

Antibiotics
Although gastroenteritis is often caused by infection it rarely needs treatment with antibiotics and then only if the nature of the germ has been established in the laboratory. Ironically for most gut germs, antibiotics seem to delay the time it takes for the germ to disappear from the system.

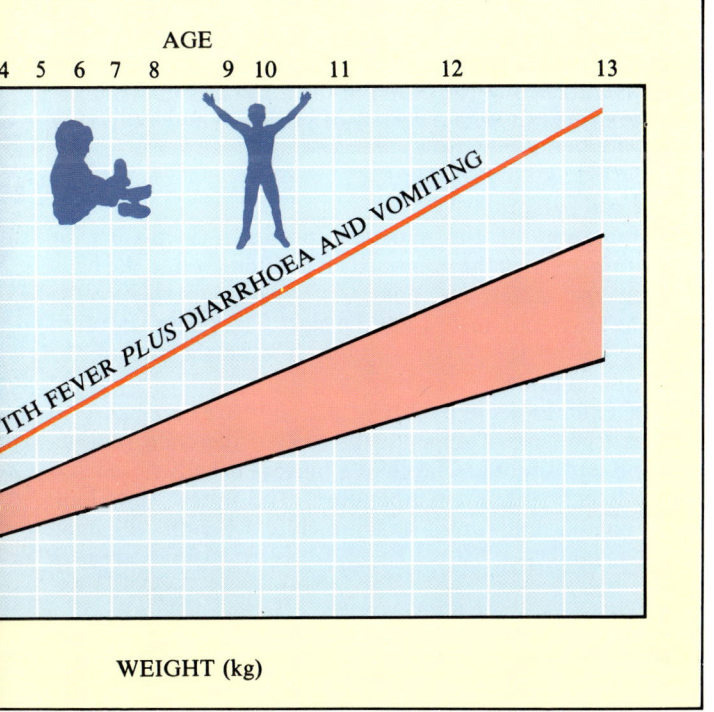

Prevention
Be very careful about preparing food and washing hands, especially after going to the toilet or changing nappies.

Gastroenteritis is usually caused by viruses and is difficult to prevent, but a lot of food poisoning is caused by food contaminated by bacteria and this can be combated by following a few simple rules.

Heat kills bacteria so food taken from the deep freeze should be thoroughly thawed and then well cooked. Beware of thick joints of meat which take surprisingly long to thaw and cook right through to the middle of the bone. Store food properly in a fridge. If meals such as cooked meat are left out in the warm, the bacteria can flourish.

If someone in the family goes down with tummy trouble, do some detective work to see if the cause can be traced. If you suspect one particular item of food it may be possible for the doctor to identify the germ in it. In this way, other members of the family may be able to avoid the problem.

Appendicitis

This condition is very rare before the age of one because of the shape and size of the appendix in babies. The appendix itself is attached to the bowel in the lower right part of the abdomen. It can lie in a variety of positions and looks very much like an earthworm.

Signs and symptoms
Inflammation of the appendix produces a mixture of symptoms. When the pain starts it is often around the belly button and comes and goes. As it gets more severe the patient may start to feel and be sick. The pain then often moves to the lower right abdomen over the site of the appendix and becomes constant.

The child looks in pain. Not many doctors are called to visit a true case of appendicitis to find the child running around and smiling. The child's pulse is usually raised and there is very often a temperature. The tongue may look very coated and furred and the child's breath will smell unpleasant.

Treatment
If you suspect this condition, contact the doctor. The treatment is surgical removal of the appendix. Do not hesitate if you are worried about appendicitis. You will see

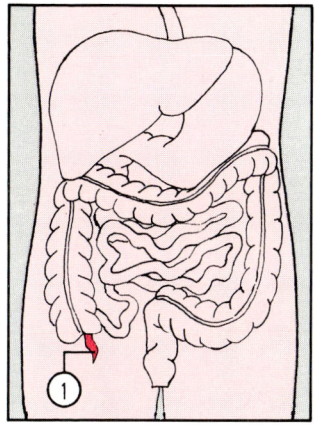

The appendix is a small appendage which lies on the right hand side of the large intestine.

it in the stages when it is important to diagnose early, yet many of the symptoms are not obvious. Delay may lead to perforation (when the appendix ruptures) and this results in peritonitis (inflammation of the membrane which surrounds the internal organs of the abdomen).

Many children do not complain of these typical signs and symptoms and this course of events may not occur. Appendicitis is not always easy to detect. Even surgeons (who usually see the patients when it is obvious!) sometimes have to operate to see what the problem is. Often it is only by looking at the appendix that you can tell if it is the cause of the belly ache.

Mesenteric adonitis

This cause of tummy ache is often one of the illnesses which is difficult to distinguish from acute appendicitis. The problem arises because during an infection elsewhere, perhaps in the ear, nose or throat, the glands in the mesentery swell up. The mesentery is a membrane within the abdominal cavity. It contains lymph glands which are similar to the others elsewhere in the body.

Because of where they are situated the glands are impossible to feel making it impossible to diagnose until the child has an operation to rule out suspected appendicitis. When this happens the surgeon finds a normal appendix but firm pink lymph glands in the mesentery. Hopefully the child will not get as far as having an operation. The symptoms usually settle in a few days though the original infection may well need treatment.

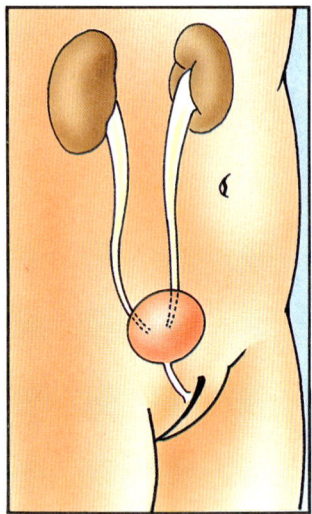

Girls are more prone to bladder and kidney infections than boys because the tube leading from the bladder to the outside (urethra) is shorter and infection can enter the bladder more easily.

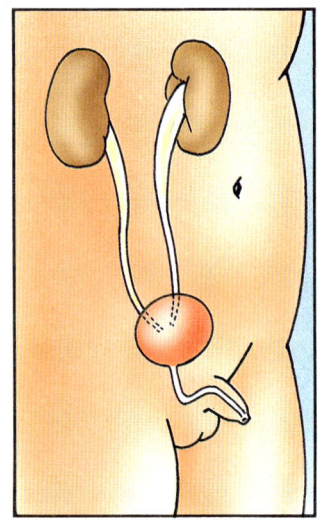

Kidney infection

An infection in the urine producing system can cause belly ache. This is much more common in girls than boys. If the infection is in the bladder the child complains of stinging and of having to go the toilet more often than usual. If the infection is higher up in the kidney then the abdomen itself will be genuinely tender in the side or sides affected.

Urinary infection may not at first be the obvious cause of an illness, so as a general rule any child with an unexplained illness, perhaps associated with a temperature, should have the urine checked.

If you suspect such an infection then let the doctor see the patient and have available a urine sample. This should be as fresh as possible. Normal urine left standing in a bottle for hours may go cloudy. (It may also go cloudy if put immediately into a cool bottle.)

To sterilize a jar, put it into cold water, bring the water to the boil and allow it to boil for ten minutes. Let the jar cool before putting in the sample.

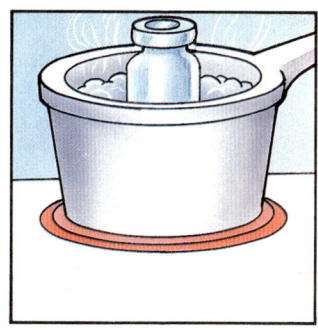

Collecting a sample

Collect the urine in a clean container such as a well washed bottle. Ideally it should go straight from the bladder into this container. This is easier said than done. If the child is old enough to cooperate the first part of the stream should be thrown away and the middle of the stream caught (a midstream urine sample, or MSU). In boys the urine should not come into contact with the foreskin so gently hold it back for the sample.

With a baby it is sometimes possible to predict when the bladder is going to be emptied, for example on waking or at a particular nappy change or feed. Almost all babies urinate if you stroke the inside of their thighs or tap their tummies for a minute or two just above the bone between the top of the legs.

Let the doctor have your best effort at collection. It will help decide if kidney infection is the problem, and what is the best treatment.

Blockage of the intestine

This is very rare but always serious. It can happen in almost any part of the abdomen and can partially or completely block off the bowel, thus the symptoms and signs may vary a little.

Complete blockage

● The child suffers with an increasingly severe colicky bellyache.
● The blockage stops things passing through so the child appears to be constipated. This causes problems the other end and food may be vomited back.
● The abdomen swells up.

Get medical help as quickly as possible if you suspect any other form of blockage.

Unexplained tummy ache

A lot of children have tummy aches which have no obvious physical cause. This does not mean that it is any less painful or distressing for the child and he or she will need just as much sympathy and tender loving care.

You don't have to be a parent for too long to realize that there is quite an obvious link between stress and anxiety and tummy ache. Rather vague tummy ache is quite common in some children at times such as going to school. It may get better during the day and disappear at weekends. Sometimes a child can be quite ill with unexplained tummy ache which may be accompanied by vomiting. Many children get tummy ache when they travel.

Also there is the rather vague term of abdominal migraine which speaks for itself. Just as adults get migraine-type headaches, it appears that children can suffer in a similar way from belly ache. A great number of children with unexplained abdominal pain go on to develop migraine as adults, particularly if their parents are migraine sufferers. The exclusion of chocolate, oranges or cheese may make a difference (see also page 70).

What to do
● Try to understand any pressures that the child is under.
● Help your child to relax. The type of reassurance needed is obviously different from the sort that you would give to an adult but try to make your child understand that coming top in the class isn't the be all and end all in life. There are compensations. Children who get abdominal migraine tend to be brighter than average.

Bedwetting

There is a lot of variation in the age at which a child becomes completely dry every night. Girls tend to manage it before boys, but most children become dry between the ages of three and four. However, a lot of normal children (perhaps one in every ten) do not stop bedwetting until after they have started school.

If your child is still wetting the bed at the age of four, or if you are worried because bedwetting starts up after the child has been dry, then go and see your doctor. Take a specimen along with you. It is very important to make sure the child has not got a longstanding urine infection.

The doctor will check that there is nothing physically

wrong. (It is very rare to find a cause such as diabetes or threadworms. See page 127).

If you child has had a period without bedwetting but it starts up again, there may be an infection or a psychological cause behind the problem. The arrival of a new baby in the family is one example of the sort of upheaval in a child's life that can cause bedwetting to recur.

What to do
The most important thing is not to overreact to the irritating business of changing a wet bed every morning. You can minimize your own work by having a plastic undersheet. Just as it is equally important not to get angry, it is important also not to go over the top and reward the child unrealistically for dry nights.

At bedtime
See that the child goes to bed with an empty bladder. As well as this potty the child when you go to bed. There is no need to wake them up. Contact with the cold potty will set off a reflex action and the bladder will soon be emptied. The child will not remember anything about this in the morning.

In the daytime
You can train the child's bladder to tolerate increasing amounts of urine. Encourage the youngster to hold his or her water until used to controlling a full bladder. Without being the least bit unkind you can make the delay between wanting to go to the toilet and actually going, longer and longer. This is the sort of thing that all adults have to do if they are caught in a place where there is no toilet.

Games and other remedies
Children enjoy games associated with having a dry bed and also seeing their achievement recorded. You can design a wall calendar and perhaps mark a dry night with some sort of tick or red star. It is a mistake to promise something like a new bicycle as a reward which is quite out of proportion to the importance of bedwetting.

The doctor may decide to use drugs or one of the buzzer alarms. It's worth saying that these do not often have to be used, and the simple home remedies that have already been outlined will usually work in the end. If drugs are used, follow the instructions.

Buzzer alarms are triggered when the child starts to wet. These are not usually effective under the age of six because the child will not know what to do if woken up anyway. Make sure that they work properly and don't become just another source of irritation to the rest of the household.

Bedwetting is not a serious childhood problem. Nearly all children eventually become dry. Undue worry about it usually creates tension and anxiety which puts off the day, or rather the night, when bedwetting is finally overcome.

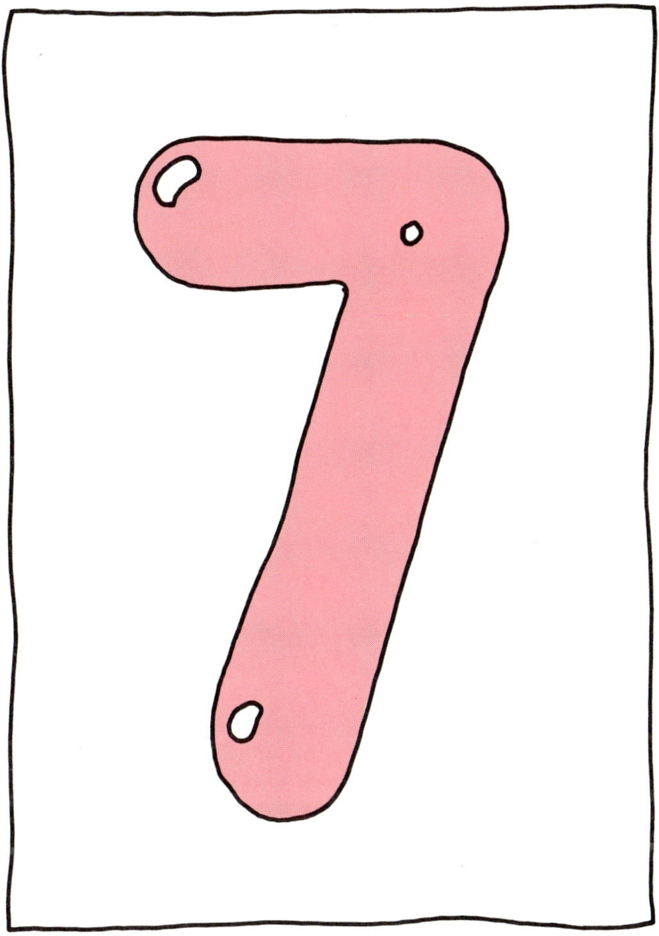

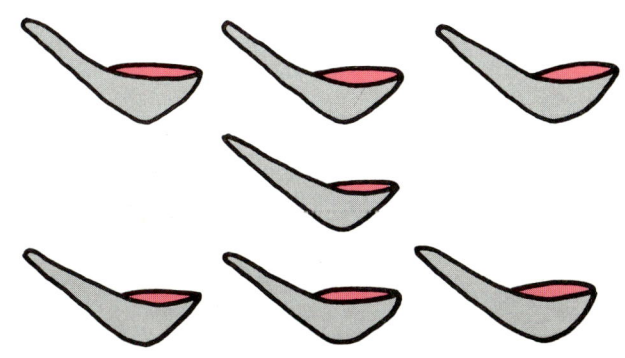

Skin trouble

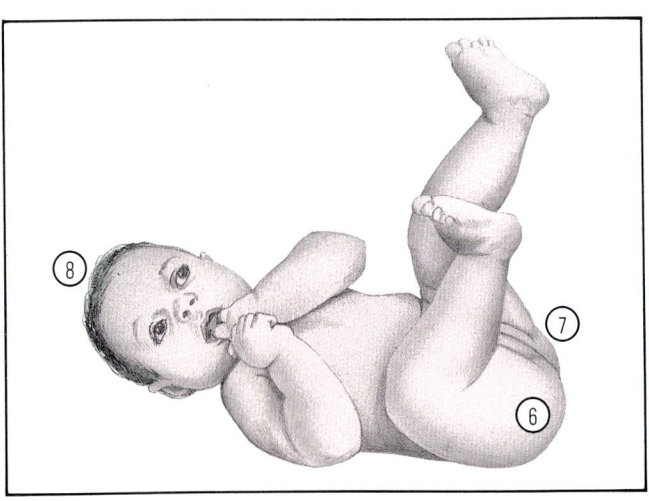

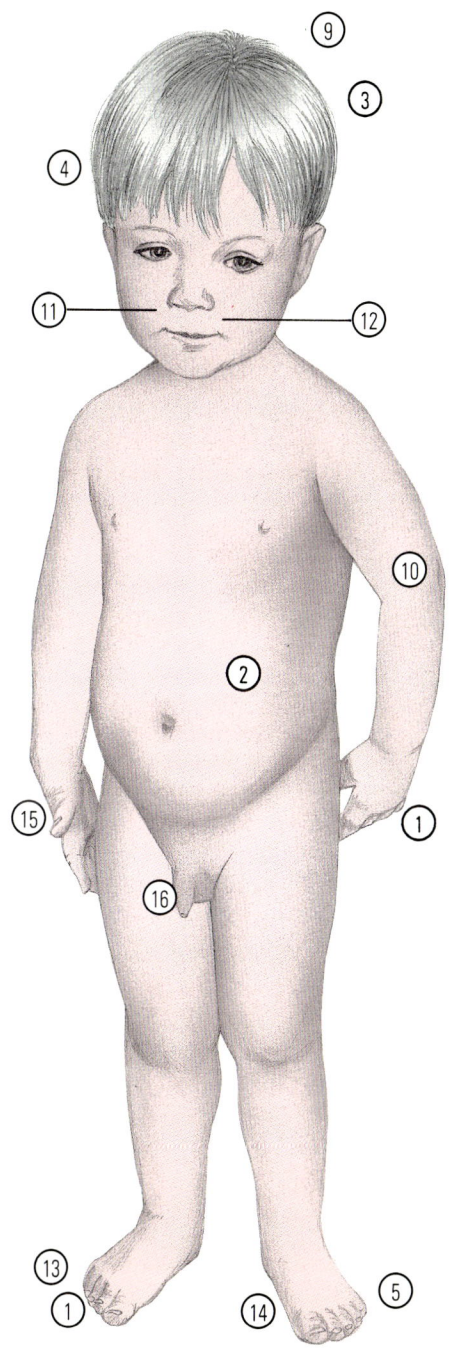

Skin trouble

Warts and verrucae

A wart is a benign skin lump caused by a virus. A verruca is a wart on the sole of the foot which the weight of the body has pushed flat or inwards. The virus is infectious and is spread in places like swimming pools, bathrooms and school gymnasiums where a child is barefoot and the virus can invade the skin. Warts and verrucae are never serious but cause a great deal of worry to parents and schools. It is understandable that teachers do not want children with verrucae to spread them around.

Is it a verruca?
Verrucae are distinguished from warts because they are on the weight-bearing areas of the foot, have a slightly darker colour than the surrounding skin and have a dark spot in the centre. They are often slightly tender which is usually the reason they are noticed in the first place.

Home care
It is important to know that warts eventually go on their own. This may account for stories of miracle cures. There is, however, scientific evidence to suggest that if a child really believes that a wart will disappear then it will. This power of suggestion can be used by the traditional method of buying the wart. Offer the child 10p (or whatever you think it's worth!), and say that if it hasn't gone within the month, then you want your money back.

There are medicines that can be bought at the chemist which chemically break down the wart. Follow the instructions for usage and be sure to cover the wart after the ointment is applied so that surrounding, healthy skin isn't damaged.

Treatment
If the wart is well-established and causing problems or concern go and see the doctor. The doctor may well recommend other treatments which can be tried if those outlined above fail. A wart can be frozen off with liquid nitrogen or scraped off after the area has been anaesthetized.

Prevention
It is important to try and stop the spread of these irritating viruses. If your child has verrucae you should buy some sort of rubber footwear for swimming.

Ringworm

A misleading word which is actually a fungal infection. It is called this because it usually spreads outwards in a ring. There are various types but the area most commonly infected in children is the skin. It may also affect the scalp, hair or nails. Ringworm is generally passed from person to person but can also be caught from animals such as dogs, cats, horses and cows.

General measures to stop ringworm spreading
- Have suspect pets checked by the vet.
- Discourage the sharing of combs, towels, shoes and brushes when ringworm is about. These are sensible measures in childhood at all times.

Ringworm of the body and scalp

This produces a circular irritating rash which slowly enlarges like a ring of fire. The edge of the rash is raised in small bumps and as it grows so the inside heals. If it affects the scalp it may cause bald patches. It can be mistaken for a patch of eczema. Consult a doctor who will prescibe anti-fungal treatment to clear it.

Athlete's foot
Athlete's foot is a fungal infection of the foot. It is common, not serious and easily cleared up if you treat the child's foot properly. It is called athlete's foot because it is acquired in showers, gymnasiums and changing rooms and athletes are more likely to have moisture between the toes, either from sweat or inadequate drying. Fungi need moisture to grow.

Signs and symptoms
The fungus grows and affects the skin between the toes, particularly the area between the fourth and fifth (little) toe. The skin becomes white, soggy and swollen.

As the fungus grows in these areas the feet can become smelly and the skin splits. In bad cases the skin underneath is red, raw and painful. It usually affects both feet.

Home treatment
The mainstay of treatment is to keep a child's feet as clean and dry as possible. People who live in the tropics and walk barefoot are rarely troubled by athlete's foot. If air

can circulate between the toes, the fungus finds it very difficult to grow. Obviously children have to wear socks and shoes at school, but buy cotton socks in preference to nylon ones and have sandals for them to wear in the summer. Let them go barefoot whenever possible.

Keep your child's washing separate because the fungus is easily spread. This is how your child caught it in the first place.

Anti-fungal preparations come as creams, ointments or powder to use on the feet. You can buy these at the chemist or get them from the doctor. Use them as advised and in conjunction with good foot care. There is little point in applying them if the child continues to have sweaty feet imprisoned in nylon socks and tight shoes. It is important that you use the cream, ointment or powder for at least a week after the symptoms have disappeared because the developing stages of the fungus can stay active in the skin for a while.

Molluscum contagiosum

This is another viral skin condition. The spots are small, round, waxy and often have a dimple in the centre. These pearl-like spots, like warts, are spread by contact. It is more common in eczematous skin.

With any sort of changing skin lump it is best to get a medical opinion. Molluscum contagiosum is easily treated once you know what it is. The doctor will show you how to scrape it off the skin.

Headlice

Headlice are small, flat, wingless insects that are a dull, brown-greyish colour. They live by sucking blood from the scalp and lay eggs which they attach to the base of the hair. These eggs hatch between two days and two weeks afterwards. They spread from person to person by direct contact and also from things such as combs, towels and hats.

How to spot them
The symptoms are actually easier to spot! A child with headlice will have an itchy scalp as a result of the insects feeding.

Look for them. They're not that easy to find, but the best areas to look are behind the ears and at the back of the scalp. Their eggs (nits) are slightly easier to see and are

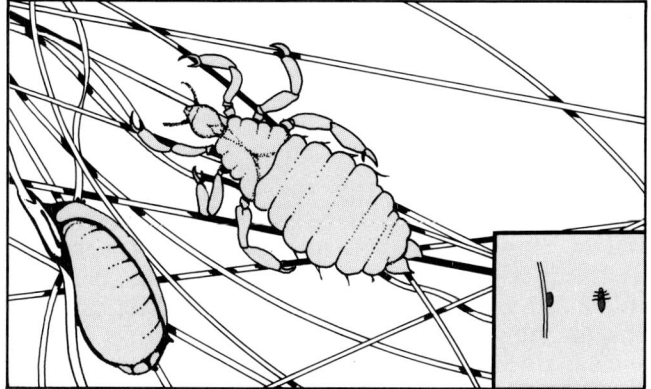

A nit (left) is the egg of the head louse (right).

small, oval and shiny yellow in colour. You may see the tiny white case left after the egg has hatched still attached to a strand of hair. It may look like dandruff or flaky skin but it won't brush away. Alternatively, ask your child to lean over a piece of white paper or sheet and vigorously brush through the hair. The dislodged lice will show up clearly against the white.

Treatment
Headlice are more common in girls, probably because they often have long hair. With a little practise (and the pictures in this book), you should be able to spot the problem as soon as it starts. Treat with a special lotion which can be bought from a chemist and follow this up with frequent combing of the child's hair. Combing has the effect of knocking off the legs of the headlice so they are unable to grip the hair. Do it regularly and their numbers will gradually diminish making this one of the best and easiest treatments. It is recommended that the whole family is treated to ensure that the headlice are completely eliminated. Combing the hair with a fine-tooth comb (available from the chemist) scrapes the nits off the hairs to which they stick very firmly.

Prevention
It is very difficult to prevent headlice and normal, healthy, clean children catch them so there is nothing to be ashamed about. Simply keep checking your children's hair regularly.

Nappy rash

Nappy rash is a common skin condition found in young babies who are still wearing nappies. Most mothers can recognize it easily. The skin is red and there may be white spots.

Nappy rash is caused by urine, stools and detergents coming into contact with the baby's sensitive skin. Although it occurs in a lot of children who are given the best of care, it is possible to prevent. The mainstay of treatment is to change the nappy frequently enough to ensure that urine and stools do not stay in contact with the skin for too long. Stagnant urine quickly breaks down to ammonia which is very irritant to the skin. Stools hasten this process.

Prevention and treatment
● Avoid using rubber or plastic pants if nappy rash breaks out. Most books on child care give this advice but I know from bitter experience that continuing to use them is a lot easier than changing a wet bed every night. I think the best compromise if you find plastic pants essential is to use the tie up sort rather than those with elastic around the legs and waist. These, like rubber pants, create a kind of greenhouse effect in which the rash thrives.
● Change your baby's nappy as often as possible. Ideally if a nappy rash looks like developing, leave the baby without a nappy. This isn't as difficult as it sounds. In the evenings leave the child wriggling about on a towel in a warm, draught-free room. Babies lie very still when asleep, so you can leave the nappy off then too.
● When you change the baby's nappy, make sure that the bottom is clean and dry. Deep skin folds need particular attention. Barrier creams like simple zinc and castor oil preparations are best for these areas and can be obtained without a doctor's prescription. Don't use talcum powder because this gets soggy and crusts in the skin creases.
● If you use washable nappies make sure that they are clean and free of any kind of detergent. Whatever washing powder you use, rinse the nappies out as thoroughly as you can.
● If the condition persists or gives reason for concern go and see the doctor. He will probably give the sort of general advice set out above or if there is any sign of infection (see Thrush below) or eczema he will prescribe a special cream to deal with it. Use it as the doctor directs.

Dandruff

Skin cells are continually shed from the surface of the body. This natural, normal process is best seen on the scalp. It causes trouble only for those with greasy skin and for those who seem to shed dead skin faster than average. Over half of us suffer from this at some time or other. Dandruff is harmless and not contagious.

There is no cure for dandruff as it is not a disease. However it can be controlled so that it does not cause worry to the child. As children get older they become understandably sensitive about the flakes of skin and the teasing dandruff can bring.

Control
1. Wash the child's hair three times a week with baby shampoo. There are medicated shampoos which can be used according to their instructions but with care and only occasionally.
2. When the condition is under control it can be kept that way by regular washing with baby shampoo. Do not try and massage the dandruff away. This stimulates the skin and can make things worse.

Thrush

Thrush is a fungal (candida) infection. The organism naturally lives in the bowels of all of us and is usually kept under control by our bacteria. If the balance between the two changes — often because a course of antibiotics has killed the good bacteria as well as the ones which make you ill — then thrush can grow excessively and become a problem.

It may produce painful, white patches in the mouth. Sometimes it causes problems at the other end of the intestinal tract and may complicate a nappy rash. A medicine is available from the doctor to clear thrush. It comes in a variety of forms such as cream, gel, spray, lotion or powder depending on where is affected.

Cradle cap

This thick, yellow-brown crusting on the scalp of babies under the age of two may appear in patches or affect the whole scalp. It often crops up over the fontanelle at the

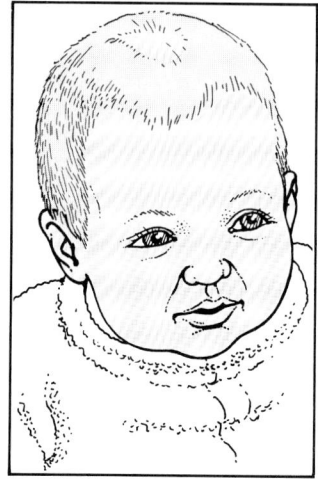

The fontanelle is a gap where the bones of the skull have not fully closed. It is covered by a tough membrane and although some parents are anxious about touching this area, no amount of washing can damage the brain underneath.

front of the head. This soft area may not get the necessary shampooing because a parent is under the mistaken belief that the baby's brain might get damaged. Often sufferers simply have a more than average greasy skin.

Treatment
In mild cases the scales will brush off and regular brushing may help prevent the problem. You can soften the scales by gently rubbing in baby oil and leaving overnight. The scales may then wash or brush off easily.

If cradle cap is more severe, and the skin itself appears inflamed and red seek the advice of your doctor or health visitor. Regular shampoos may fail to help at this stage. Medicated shampoos are available which if applied correctly clear the cradle cap up in a few days. Use them as directed. They are often best put on at night and then washed off as a shampoo in the morning.

Prevention
● Brush the hair regularly.
● Wash the baby's hair regularly and thoroughly.

Eczema

Eczema is an extremely itchy, dry skin condition. It affects various parts of the body, although some areas, like the backs of the knees, behind the ears and in the creases of the elbows are characteristic. It is not infectious and the child must not be made to feel like a leper. If the skin gets scratched and red raw and starts to weep then it can get infected.

The causes of eczema are not fully understood. Sometimes the term dermatitis is used instead. This literally means inflammation of the skin.

Atopic eczema

This is the most common form of the condition in children. It doesn't usually start until the child is three or four months old. There are often others in the family with allergic conditions such as asthma and hayfever. The child may grow out of the eczema, but be left with these other forms of allergy. Although the causes (and there are probably many) are not fully understood, stress and an emotional upset can trigger things off or make them worse if they are already present.

The rash often begins on the cheeks and can spread anywhere, but particularly to the body creases mentioned above.

There is as yet no certain cure for all types of eczema. It is important to see a doctor so that the diagnosis can be confirmed. Some rashes are not serious and need no treatment but seborrhoeic eczema in particular can be helped quickly by treatment.

Treatment

These aim to reduce the symptoms of eczema either by softening the skin, or by relieving the itchiness.

1. **Moisturizers**

The child's skin should be kept clean and soft and must be prevented from drying out. There are a number of creams and oils to do this. Some can be put into the bath water. (Beware. They can make children as slippery as a bar of soap!) These are **not** steroid creams. They aim to keep a dry skin moist.

2. **Steroid Creams and Ointments**

These anti-inflammatory preparations can produce a dramatic improvement in symptoms. There are now some available without prescription. They must be used with great care in children as prolonged use can damage the skin, especially of the face. Do not put them on the face without medical advice.

Always ask what is in a cream or ointment you are given. There are many different preparations around both with and without steroids. Those with steroids vary a great deal in strength. Use the weakest ones that will control the condition at the time. You can switch to a lower strength as the inflammation subsides.

3. Antihistamines
These medicines can help control itchiness. They are particularly helpful at night because they also often make children sleepy.

Home care
A number of precautions can be taken at home to help children cope with the discomfort of eczema.

1. Foods
Food does seem to play a part in eczema, although no one is sure exactly what. Do not put your child on any kind of food exclusion diet without medical advice.

Breast feed the child for the first six months if possible. When you wean the child onto other foods watch carefully for any reaction to a particular food. Dairy products, chocolate, eggs, fish, wheat, and certain colourings such as Tartrazine (yellow) and preservatives often come under suspicion.

2. Clothes
Put the child in cotton clothes. Wool and nylon can make the irritation worse. Change nappies quickly once they are soiled. Soft washable terry nappies are often better than disposable ones for children with eczema. Make sure they are well washed of any detergent. Avoid biological detergents. If at all possible do not use plastic pants when the skin is sore.

Bed clothes should be chosen with care. Wool, feather and down can make eczema worse. Cotton is a good material for pillow and duvet covers. The bedroom should be kept as free of dust as possible.

3. General skin care
Keep the skin clean and beware of it drying out. Pat it dry after a bath and use the moisturizers as above. Fingernails should be kept short and clean for obvious reasons. Most soaps which are fine for normal skin are too drying and

irritating for eczema sufferers and bubble baths which contain detergents should be avoided. Ask your doctor for advice about what to use.

4. Detective work
You may find that there are other factors which cause the eczema to flare up. Many parents keep a diary and are able to track down trigger factors such as certain animals, a special time or place, a season, or even an event which a sensitive child finds upsetting or stressful.

5. National Eczema Society (see Useful Addresses, page 156). It can be helpful to meet other families with eczema. You can exchange views and experiences. It helps to know to know you are not alone.

Although some eczema settles quickly with treatment it may become troublesome and chronic and require much greater care, devotion and hard work. Fortunately it usually improves as children get older.

Seborrhoeic eczema
This is a different sort of eczema. It tends to clear quickly and does not run in allergic families. It affects parts of the body where there are seborrhoeic (grease producing) glands. It can be divided up as follows:

1. **Blepharitis.** The skin at the edge of the eyelids becomes inflamed. The eyelashes appear to have dandruff, and the lids are red and scaly.

2. **Otitis externa.** This affects the lining of the outer ear canal (see page 77).

3. Severe form of **cradle cap** (see above). The crusts of simple cradle cap have a sore red itchy scalp underneath. Seborrhoeic dermatitis can also spread to other parts of the body.

Impetigo
A bacterial skin infection which usually starts when the skin is broken in some way. The face and hands are the areas most often affected. It may follow cold sores or when conditions such as ezcema cause the skin to be

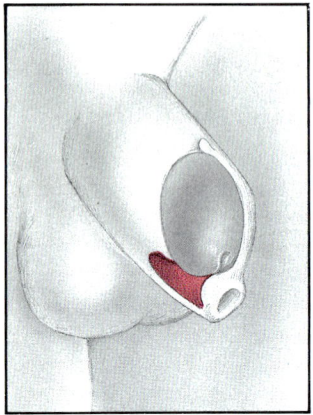

The frenulum attaches the foreskin to the shaft of the penis. In a young boy it is not possible to fully retract the foreskin, and although good hygiene is important, more harm than good is done by forcing back the foreskin which may tear the frenulum and cause troublesome scarring.

scratched. It is very infectious and can spread to other parts of the body, and also to other children.

It usually clears quickly when antibiotic creams are applied. Sometimes antibiotics by mouth are necessary. Encourage the child not to touch impetigo. Keep the skin as clean and dry as possible. Activities such as picking the nose help it spread.

Balanitis

This is inflammation of the tip of the penis. If the boy is still in nappies it may be part of a nappy rash. After the age of about five it should be possible to roll the child's foreskin back. Sometimes if it is tight and cannot be rolled back for washing the area can get inflamed.

If this happens the end of the penis becomes red and painful and there may be a yellow discharge. It will not be possible to draw the foreskin back at this stage, so do not try.

Contact the doctor. An antibiotic will clear up the acute phase.

Prevention
Good hygiene is the key to stopping it happening again. It may be part of a nappy rash (see page 118).

Up until the age of about five the foreskin is part of the bud-like tip of the penis. Before this time it is a mistake to try and force it back. Some doctors suggest trying to coax it back after the age of four when your son is relaxed and warm in the bath, others simply say let nature take its course. Once you see the foreskin naturally beginning to separate from the end of the penis (the glans) then get the child used to the idea that this part of the body needs to be kept clean. Wash under the foreskin regularly.

Circumcision for medical rather than religious reasons is rarely necessary if the foreskin is going back by the time the boy is eight. Consult the doctor if the foreskin will not do this or if urine does not pass out in a good straight flow. If the foreskin is too tight the stream of urine will shoot out at all angles and the foreskin will balloon out.

Chilblains

Some children are over-sensitive to the cold. This produces painful, red, itchy areas on the fingers, toes, nose and ears called chilblains. There is no ideal cure, simply keep the child well wrapped-up and warm in cold weather. It helps to keep the feet dry and change the socks every couple of days. It is useful to have two pairs of shoes so that one can be drying out while the others are being worn.

If chilblains cause continuing problems to the child then go and see the doctor or pharmacist. There may be a cream or ointment that can be put onto the skin to ease the symptoms.

Cold sores

These are sores, usually on the face around the mouth or nose, that are produced by the herpes simplex virus.

They can be very unpleasant, especially if they become recurrent. The virus becomes active when the child gets run down for any reason, such as after a cold. Sunlight also seems to trigger cold sores.

When the blister forms try and stop the child touching or licking the area (see Impetigo above). The sore can be dried up by applications of surgical spirit. A scab forms after about a week and comes off in the following few days.

Consult the doctor if the sores are persistent or if they erupt near the eyes. There are now creams occasionally prescribed to inactivate the herpes virus.

Herpes virus has had a bad press in recent years because of sexually-transmitted genital herpes in adults. Although the problem is similar, the problems adults have with genital herpes are not relevant to cold sores in children. The virus is, however, spread by contact so do not let a child with a cold sore kiss other children.

Boils

A boil is a bacterial infection at the root of a hair. The surrounding area becomes red hot and swollen as the yellow pus collects. If it happens around an eyelash it's called a stye (see page 88).

A boil will usually come to a head and discharge naturally after about three days. Do not squeeze them as this spreads the infection. Home treament involves helping pain and stopping the spread of the germs as the boil takes its course, so do not allow the child to touch the area. The skin can be bathed in warm water and a clean dressing placed over it. Clean the discharge away with a clean dressing as the boil bursts and healing begins.

Seek medical help if the boil does not discharge after five days. Boils near the eye pose particular dangers and medical help should be sought.

Ingrowing toenails

This painful condition happens when the growing toenail cuts into the fleshy side of the toe, usually one of the big toes. The toe can get infected causing the toe to be even more painful and red and the side of nail may also leak pus. This may need a course of antibiotics from the doctor.

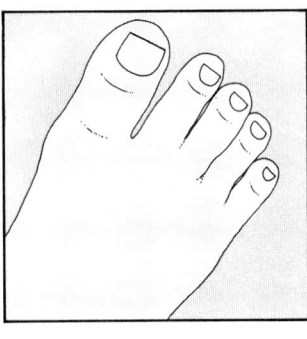

Cut toenails straight across leaving the outer edges of the nail clear of the cuticle surround.

A V-shaped cut in the centre of the nail may be enough to relieve pressure on the outer edges.

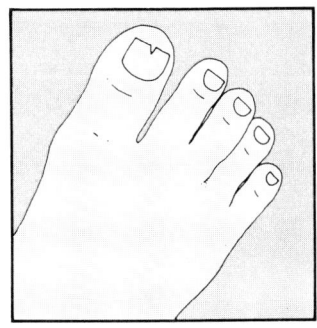

Ingrowing toenails are best prevented. Cut the toenails straight across, and not too short. Shoes and socks must fit properly and should not be too tight.

If the nail does start to grow into the flesh of the foot you may be able to nip the problem in the bud by cutting a small v-shape in the middle of the nail. This takes the pressure off the sides. Clean the nail and toe and put an antiseptic cream on the area.

If the nail continues to cause problems then seek medical aid. The toe will not heal until the nail has been sorted out and it is not advisable to poke around and do this yourself.

Scabies

Scabies is an intensely itchy skin condition caused by a mite. The female mite burrows into the skin to lay her eggs. This causes the itching which is worse at night when the child gets warm in bed. It is spread by close contact from person to person.

The burrows are only a millimetre or two long and may have a dark spot at one end. They can occasionally be seen by the naked eye but often the child's scratching has destroyed all trace of them.

The areas affected by scabies are the fingers, the front of the wrists, and around the lower abdomen and genitals where the mite burrrows into soft, thin skin. It hardly ever affects a child's head. Suspect it if other close contacts have had scabies.

Do not instantly suspect scabies if your child starts scratching. Many things cause this symptom, and the itching often seems worse in a warm bed at night.

If you are worried about scabies go and see the doctor. It is not serious and is cleared up by a special skin lotion with which all close contacts of the child must also be treated. It is important that bedding and underclothes are given a hot wash to remove all trace of the mites.

Worms

There are a variety of worms which can enter and live inside a child's body. Most are rare outside the tropics but the threadworm is very common in the United Kingdom.

Threadworms

These are passed on when the small eggs are swallowed. They hatch out in the intestines and grow into the adult, white thread-like worms which are up to half an inch long. The cycle continues when the female comes out of the back passage at night to lay more eggs. This causes intense itching, and very occasionally is the cause of bedwetting in a child.

The eggs are then in a position to get passed on again. Perhaps the child scratches his or her bottom and the eggs lodge under the nails or simply on the thumb when it gets sucked. They may be passed on to other children simply by holding hands at games.

Suspect threadworms if the child is scratching the bottom at night. You can look for the female worm around the anus, or in the child's stool. It will probably be moving like a piece of white cotton.

Treatment
1. Two doses of a medicine such as Pripsen will kill the worms. Take the medicine as prescribed. It is important that all the family is treated (including the father).
2. To stop the worms getting back again, children should be made to wash their hands after going to the toilet. Fingernails should be kept short and clean.

Threadworms are an occupational hazard of being young. Anyone can catch them and they are nothing to be ashamed about. The treatment is fast and if taken correctly always works, although reinfection is common.

Roundworm
This is very rare. The worm is like a white earthworm, and is usually picked up abroad in the tropics. Look out for them in the stools. They are a very rare cause of a child failing to thrive. Treatment is usually with a similar drug as for threadworms.

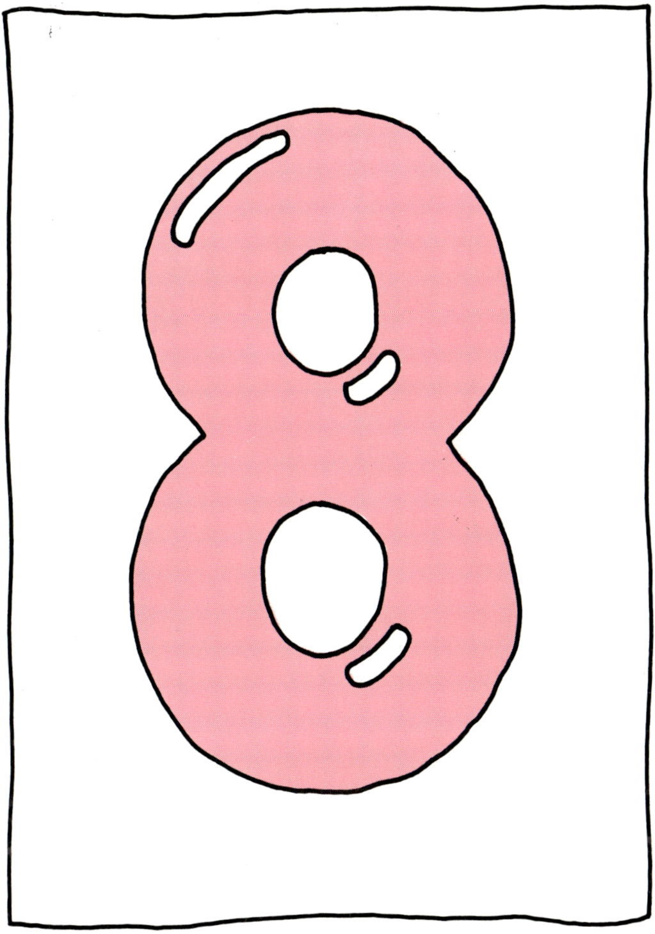

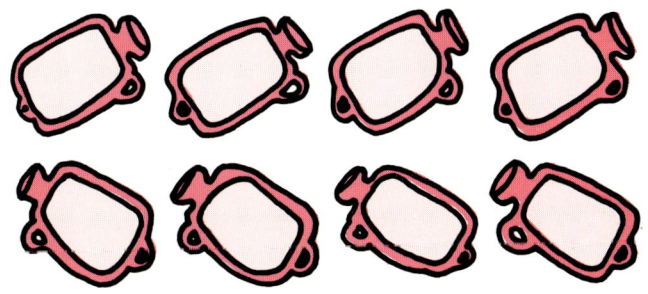

Safe home

1. Put vertical bars on upstairs windows or childproof locks. Horizontal bars may be used as a climbing frame.

2. Keep all cosmetics, medicines (e.g. iron tablets taken during pregnancy) and electrical appliances such as hairdryers out of reach.

3. Have cupboards that can be pushed open from the inside in case the child gets shut in.

4. Have stable furniture that will not topple over if used to climb on.

5. Do not leave an electric blanket on in an unattended room.

6. The mantlepiece above the fire should be clear of any item that may attract child's interest.

7. Attach fireguard to wall.

8. Lock older children's toys away.

9. Have safety glass in door.

10. Keep safety covers on all electrical plugs which are within reach.

11. Alternatively have plugs which children cannot reach.

12. Straps should be worn at all times in the high chair.

13. Avoid tablecloths which may be pulled down along with scalding cups.

14. Keep plastic bags and household cleaning agents in a cupboard out of reach.

15. Alternatively keep the cupboards locked.

16. Do not leave hot cups of tea or coffee within reach.

17. Keep a guard around the cooker at all times.

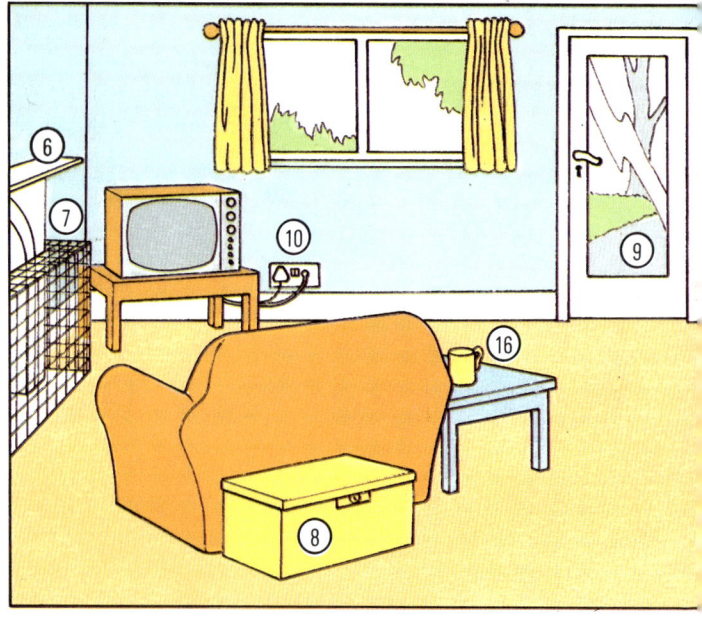

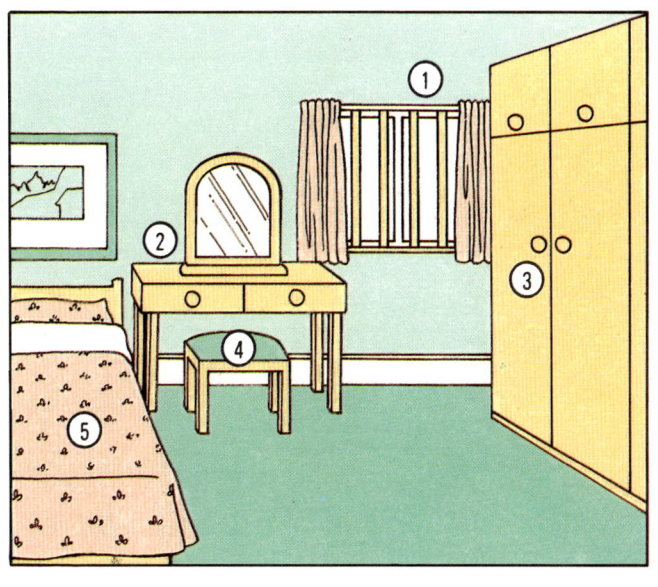

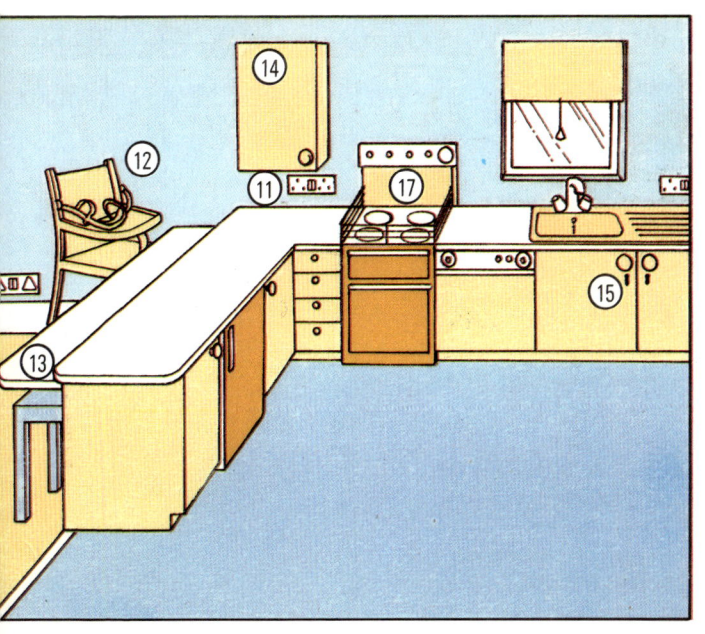

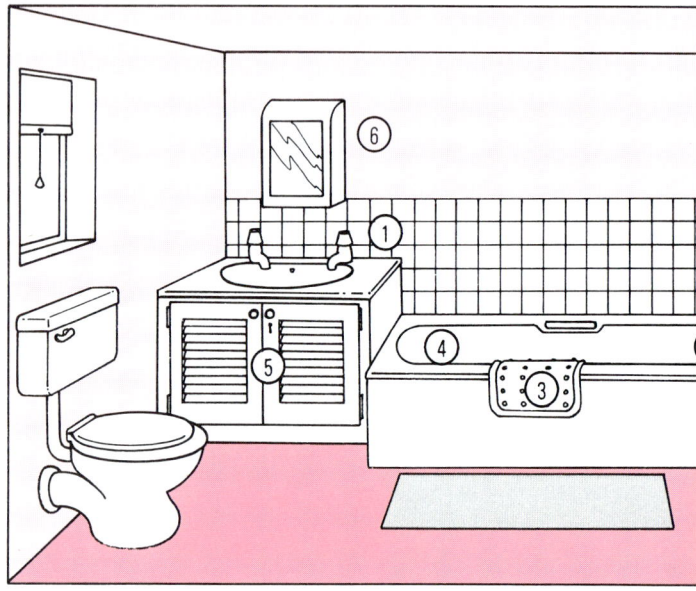

1. Keep water temperature low enough not to scald.

2. Never run the hot water into the bath first. Run both taps or the cold first.

3. Use a non-slip mat, even for older children.

4. Never leave children unattended at bathtime.

5. Lock away bathroom cleaners.

6. Keep all medicines out of reach.

7. Make sure the lock on the bathroom door cannot be reached by a child.

8. A safety gate at the top of the stairs is essential, another at the foot is advisable.

9. Children must learn never to eat anything they find in the garden. Laburnum pods for example, can be lethal.

10. Keep garden equipment in good repair. Soft grass is the safest material to fall off onto.

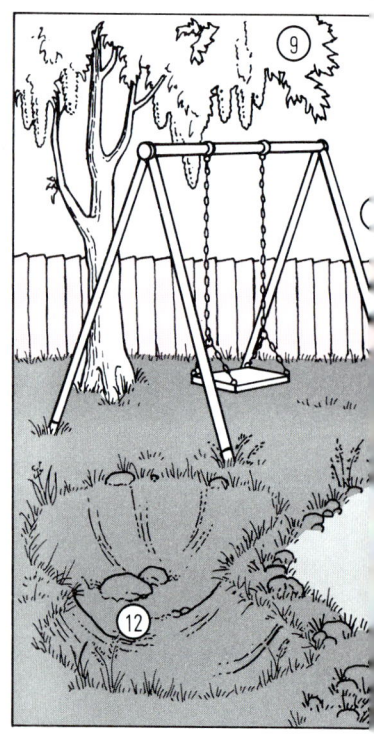

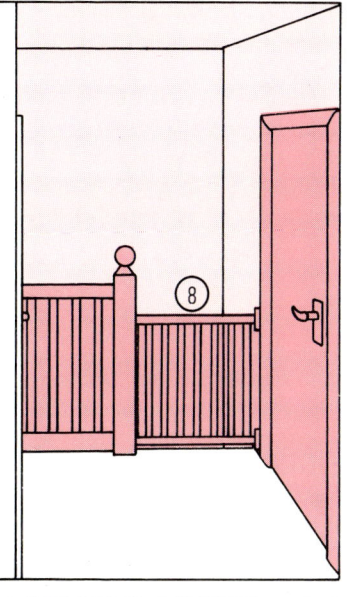

11. Secure all garden gates.
12. Drain ponds. A child can drown in a few inches of water.
13. Secure the tops of waterbutts.
14. Padlock garden shed and garage.
15. Keep chemicals and weedkillers clearly marked in their own bottles locked away.
16. If applying weedkillers to paths, do it when children are not around. Use chemicals which are neutralized on contact with earth. Small children will put gravel and stones in their mouths.

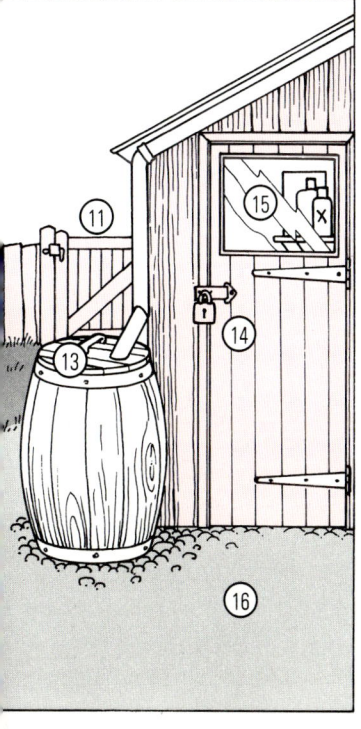

Accidents

Accidents are the greatest cause of death and disablement in childhood and about half of these are the result of road accidents.

Some accidents are unavoidable but a great many are unnecessary. Seat belts for children in the back of cars, for example, would prevent a great many of these deaths and there are a number of avoidable dangers in the house and garden which still account for a large proportion of accidents each year.

Choking

A child chokes for two different reasons; either because something is lodged in the tube leading to the stomach (the oesophagus) or because it is lodged in the tube leading to the lungs (the bronchus). The oesophagus is soft and flexible, but the trachea is unyieldingly restricted by rings of cartilage and becomes narrower as it progresses. Dangerous choking is due to a blockage of the airway anywhere between the mouth and lungs. That may be at the back of the mouth, which makes the child gag. It is often possible to slide a finger a little way down the throat and hook the lump out. This is far less distressing for a child than being turned upside down and thumped between the shoulder blades.

However, if something has lodged in the windpipe and is stopping the child from breathing, it must be dislodged as quickly as possible otherwise the child could die within a few minutes. It is not that difficult to do if you think clearly and act quickly.

Action

For a baby
The baby's head must be lower than its chest, so hold him or her upside down by the feet, or lay head down over your knees. Bang hard four times between the shoulder blades. The aim is to knock the wind out of the lungs without breaking the springy rib cage. Any inhaled foreign body like a toy should shoot out of the mouth.

For an older child
You will not be able to hold him or her upside down, so lay the child head down over your knee or a chair, and again bang between the shoulder blades four times.

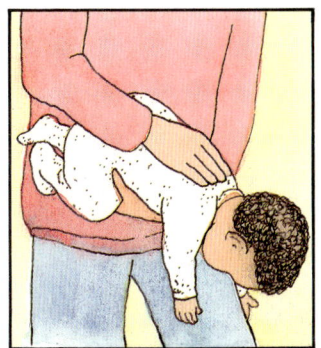

A small baby can be held upside down and banged between the shoulder blades to dislodge something from the windpipe. An older child should be laid head down across a lap.

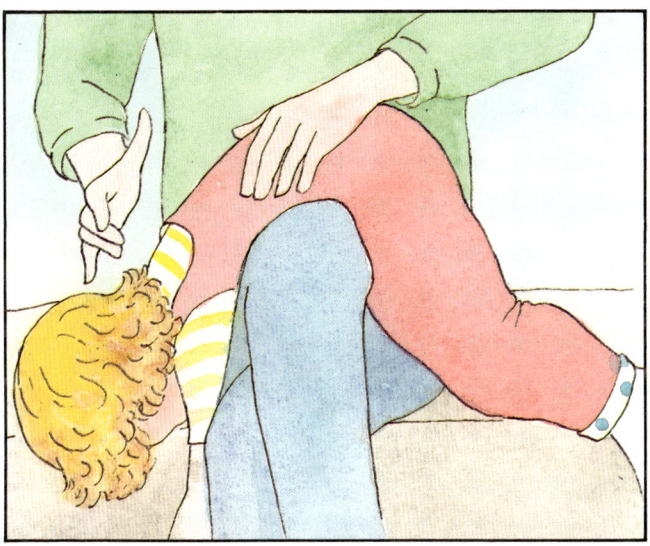

Prevention

It is difficult to stop children putting things in their mouths, but a few general rules can minimize the risks.

● Never give a small child peanuts because they can get inhaled right down into the lungs. They also cause other problems like chest infections which do not settle with the usual treatment.

● Keep older children's toys, such as marbles, out of reach of younger brothers and sisters. Babies between the ages of six and twelve months put everything in their mouths instinctively. Make sure they only get hold of things that cannot fit in their mouths.

Cuts and grazes

Children regularly cut and graze themselves, and most of these injuries can be treated by washing with soap and warm water and leaving them to heal under nature's dressing, the scab. Bleeding tends to clean a wound. It is impossible to get all the germs out of a cut or graze. The body's own defences will take care of these and particles of dirt will come away when the scab comes off.

If you feel a dressing would be helpful (some children love them as a kind of badge of bravery!) and to stop the child picking or knocking the wound, use something like a sterile gauze held on by some sort of tape. These are cheap, easy to put on and change, and the air can get to the wound. Remember, however, that dressings can stick to a wound and will have to be carefully peeled or soaked off. Change dressings daily to avoid this and leave the wound uncovered at night after a couple of days to allow the scab to dry hard. All in all a scab is probably the best covering for cuts and grazes.

Deeper cuts

There are certain types of cuts which should be taken more seriously and you need to assess whether you should consult the doctor. A ragged edged, dirty wound needs expert cleaning. Amateur probing may simply push infection deeper into a wound. A sharp clean cut made with a knife carries far less potential danger than a cut from a piece of glass in the vegetable patch.

Consult the doctor if you think a cut needs a stitch. This is largely a matter of common sense. Remember that it is more important that cuts on the face heal perfectly than, for example, those hidden by hair on the scalp. Another thing to consider is the site of the cut. One in an area of strain, such as a cut over the kneecap, is more likely to reopen than one on a part of the body which is not continually moving. Some cuts can be quite easily held together by adhesive strips or by dumbell-shaped plasters.

If the area of the cut seems to get more tender as the days pass, watch out for signs of infection which may develop after a day or so even in the best attended injury. The surrounding area is red and hot, and you may see yellow fluid in the wound. This needs expert attention. Deep puncture wounds are more likely to get infected than open grazes.

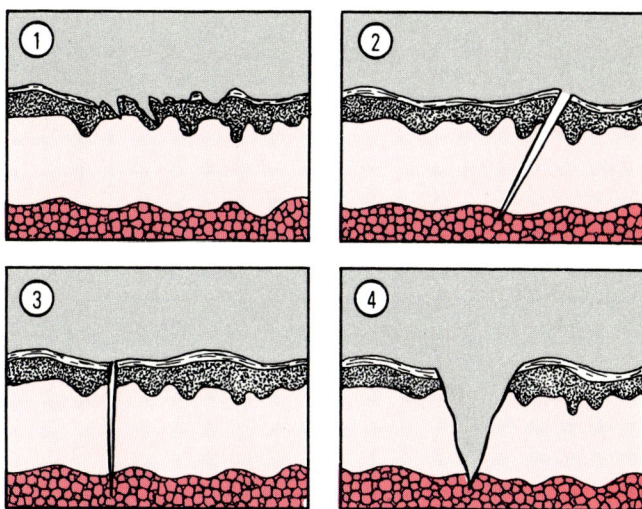

A graze (1) superficially damages the surface of the skin. A clean cut (2) is deeper but heals well but a puncture wound (3) may harbour infection because the entrance hole is closed over. If the edges of a cut are gaping (4) it may need stitches to prevent an insightly scar forming.

Bleeding

This can be very alarming, but remember that areas such as the scalp bleed heavily when cut, and a small amount of blood seems to go a long way. It is important not to panic because a child will sense this and become unnecessarily alarmed. Panic and fear make most situations more difficult to handle and control and are not helpful in a casualty.

The body has its own in-built mechanism to stop bleeding, and most small cuts will stop on their own. If the bleeding is more profuse, you can help this natural process by applying firm pressure with a clean pad, bandage or handkerchief for five to ten minutes. Alternatively, pinch the edges of the cut together. This is the length of time it takes for blood vessels to close, and for a clot to form. Once you have stopped the bleeding, do not restart it by interfering with the wound. Resist the temptation to take the pad off to see if the bleeding has stopped. If you have stopped it, it will start again when you remove the delicate clot attached to the pad. Any cleaning should be done before stopping the blood flow.

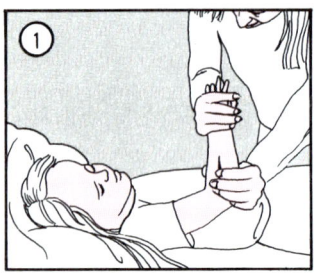

Raise a bleeding limb (1) because this will reduce the flow. If the wound is gaping (2) you can literally hold the edges together. Pressure (3) will stop even copious bleeding provided you keep it up for a full ten minutes.

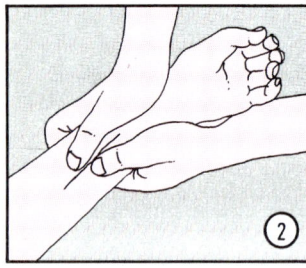

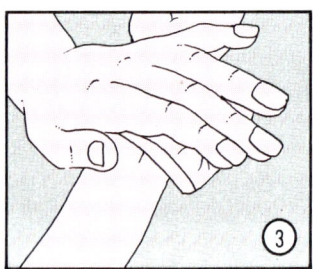

Either sit or lay the young casualty down in a comfortable position. Raise the injured area if possible. Blood is like water, it flows faster downhill than up. Some of you are, unfortunately, going to see children who are bleeding very heavily. However, direct pressure will stop even the most severe blood loss until medical help is available. (See Shock page 150).

Nosebleed
Again, do not panic! The blood may look a lot but this emergency can nearly always be dealt with quickly and simply if you follow the following steps.
1. Sit the child forward.
2. Pinch the soft part of the nose just below the bridge.
3. This must be done for ten minutes. Time it with a clock or watch. During this time the child breathes through the mouth and spits blood out into a bowl. Swallowing blood may make the child sick.
4. It will nearly always have stopped after the ten minutes if you do this correctly. It is important then not to let the child disturb the clot by sniffing or blowing the nose. This will restart the bleeding and you will need to start the process again if this happens!
5. If after ten minutes **by the clock** of continual pressure the bleeding has not stopped, call the doctor.

Tooth Socket

If the gums bleed after a tooth has either come out or been extracted then it must be stopped. Get a piece of gauze or cotton wool and place over the bleeding area. (A tampon or a tea bag is ideal for this). Ask the child to bite on it. There should be enough gauze to prevent the teeth meeting. The aim is not to fill the hole where the tooth has come out, but to increase the pressure sufficiently to stop the flow of blood.

The same rules apply as with nosebleeds. After ten minutes the bleeding should have stopped. After that it is important not to disturb the soft clot which looks like a piece of soft liver at the base of the socket.

Concussion and head injuries

Concussion occurs when a violent shaking of the brain causes a temporary loss of consciousness. It is usually the result of a bang on the head and often does not result in any major or long-term problems. However, any child who has been knocked out should be seen by a doctor and observed. Some complications only become apparent in the hours after the incident when the child appears to be recovering.

Children bang their heads an awful lot. One expert worked out that a pre-school child may fall over an average 13 times a day! In most cases they are up and playing again within minutes.

Assessing the situation

If there is a cut on the head, stop the bleeding and decide whether a doctor may need to stitch it up.

Find out if the child was knocked out. If the answer is yes, you must seek medical help. If an adult did not see what happened ask other children if your child cried and moved around immediately afterwards.

If there is no one to ask but the casualty, the following questions asked calmly will soon indicate if the child was knocked out. "Do you remember what happened? Do you remember what happened immediately before and after the accident?" (Things like hitting the floor and crying.) If there has been memory loss, the child has probably suffered a concussion.

It is important to know exactly where the head was hit. The child will tell you where it's sore; feel gently and you may be able to find a lump. The temple and over the ear are danger areas (which is why sports helmets are designed the way they are with special protection above the ears.) In this area there is an artery under the skull which is naturally stuck to the bone. This is an unfortunate piece of human design because it means the artery is much more easily broken than other blood vessels around the brain. Bumps on the forehead and back of the head tend to be less serious.

Look for any blood or clear fluid leaking from the ear. This is a serious sign because the fluid surrounding the brain may be leaking out through a crack in the skull.

Call the doctor if:

● You think a cut needs stitching (see page 136).
● The child has been knocked out, or if you are worried.
● There is a severe, persistent headache.
● The child vomits more than once.
● The child falls into an unusual sleep, for example, breathing with a strange pattern, or grunting.
● There is any unusual behaviour, or unsteady gait or awkward movements.
● You cannot easily rouse the child. Check this by giving the child a shake without actually waking him or her up. If the injury happens near bedtime, then you will have to sacrifice some sleep to keep an eye on him or her.

Resuscitation

The basic treatment for someone who appears to have died can easily be remembered, even in an emergency, by the first three letters of the alphabet.
The ABC of resuscitation is **Airway, Breathing, Circulation.**

A. Airway

Check that this is clear. There must be a clear passage from the mouth past the back of the throat and down the windpipe into the lungs. Problems usually come when the tongue slips to the back of the throat. Raise the chin and tilt the head backwards to help lift the tongue forward to unblock the airway. At the same time anything else blocking the airway such as vomit can quickly be scooped out with two fingers.

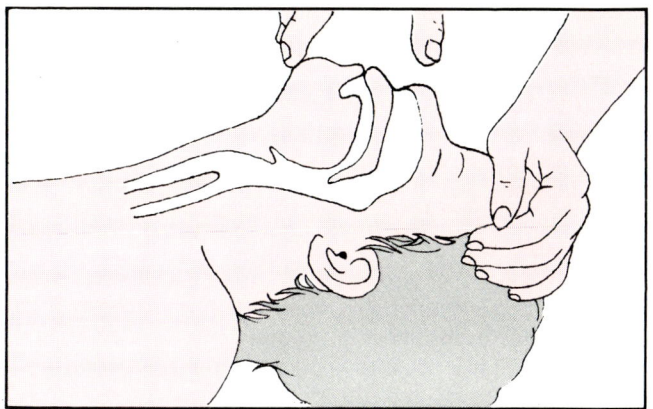

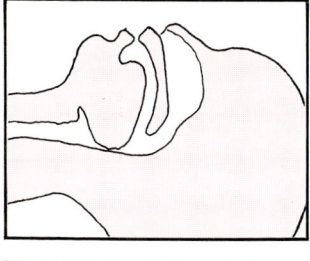

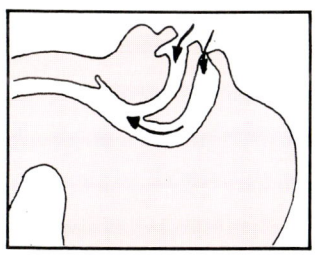

If the child is making a gargling noise, there may be something blocking the airway. Clearing out the mouth and throat may be enough to start the child breathing again.
The tongue of an unconscious child falls to the back of the throat and blocks the airway.
Raising the chin lifts the tongue forward and frees the airway.

B. Breathing

If breathing has stopped you must start it again artificially. This is the traditional mouth-to-mouth artificial respiration, more popularly called the kiss of life.

C. Circulation

If the heart has stopped you have to do the pumping for it, otherwise the mouth-to-mouth resuscitation which will be getting oxygen into the lungs is a waste of time. Blood needs to be circulating, even artificially, to take this oxygen from the lungs to the brain. Without it the brain starts to die irreversibly within minutes.

Following drowning children have recovered after long periods of resuscitation. Always keep going until you get more skilled help.

Artificial resuscitation cannot be learnt from pictures. It is easy to learn with practise, but it is not safe to practise on a healthy person or child. Go on a course and learn how to do it.

Burns and Scalds
There are a number of ways heat can damage the skin and all except very minor burns must be taken seriously.

Superficial burns are very painful. Deep extensive burns mercifully are not because the nerve endings are destroyed. There are two real dangers with burns: infection through the broken skin, and fluid loss from the circulation, and these are more severe if the blisters are popped. Both these conditions can cause the circulation to fail — this is shock.

● Dry burns are caused by touching hot objects such as stoves and cookers and also by exposure to a fierce sun.
● Wet burns or scalds are caused by steam and boiling liquids.
● Electric burns can damage the body in a number of ways. It may set clothing on fire and it may also do internal damage similar to a crush injury. Electrical burns must be taken very seriously because the extent of the damage is not always obvious to the eye. An electric shock may stop the heart and the breathing. Such a casualty needs resuscitation (see page 140).
● Friction burns are caused by sliding down ropes or from touching something revolving at high speed.
● Chemical burns result from contact with chemicals like acids and alkalis.

Action
Treatment of minor dry burns and scalds
1. Ease the pain. Run cold water from the tap over the burn for at least ten minutes. If you are away from running water immerse the burn in a bowl of cold water. Give the patient one of the paracetamol mixtures.
2. Keep the burn clean. If a dressing is necessary use one that is clean and dry. Do not prick blisters or put anthing like butter on the burn. Protect them from being rubbed and bursting. If blisters do burst cover them with a clean dressing. A clean, ironed tea towel is often the most sterile item in the average home.

Treatment of electrical burns
1. Switch off the electical current if possible. If this is not possible break the contact with something wooden like a broom handle that will not conduct the current to you.
2. Check that the child is still breathing and the heart is still beating. Start resuscitation if necessasry.
3. Treat as a serious burn and call for expert help immediately.

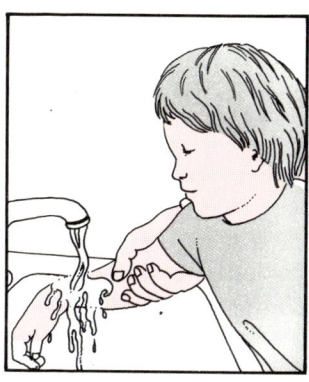

If a caustic chemical comes into contact with a child's skin, slowly run water over the area for at least ten minutes to prevent further damage. Maintain the flow as you carefully remove contaminated clothing.

Treatment of chemical burns
1. Run water over the damaged area to dilute and wash away the chemical.
2. Carefully remove contaminated clothing.
3. Treat as a serious burn unless the damage is very minor and get expert help immediately.
4. If chemicals get into the eye, quickly wash under clean, running water. After irrigating it like this, cover with a clean pad and seek medical help.

Sunburn

Protect a child with a shirt over his or her bathing costume in the first few days of hot sunshine. Be especially wary if your child is red or fair-skinned.

Protective lotions and creams applied frequently do help but none offer complete protection from sunburn. The creams come in various factors depending on how much of the sun's light they filter out. (Factor 0, nil; factor 15, almost all.) Use them wisely when the child is first exposed to the sort of unaccustomed sun of a foreign holiday. Pay special attention to the nose and back of neck, and reapply after swimming.

Action for sunburn
1. Cool the red burnt areas with calamine lotion.
2. Treat blisters as above.
3. Rest the child in the shade and give him or her plenty of cold fruit drinks. Add in paracetamol mixture with this as necessary.
4. Cover the burns during the day with loose light clothes. Indoors and at night leave them exposed.
5. Treat bad sunburn as a serious burn.

When to call the doctor for sunburn
● If the child's temperature goes up over 39°C and the child is drowsy and unwell.
● Heatstroke can complicate sunburn and should be treated seriously.The body's thermostat has broken down and the skin becomes hot and dry, not hot and sweaty. The temperature may go over 40°C. In addition the pulse is rapid and the child may become drowsy and finally lapse into unconciousness. You need expert medical help.

Emergency treatment of severe burns

Wet burns
1. Lay the casualty down and if he or she is conscious give plenty of reassurance.
2. Remove burnt clothing. Cut away any clothing soaked with chemicals or boiling water but do not pull at clothing which seems stuck to the skin. It is important to do this quickly and remember too to take off anything which will become tight as the body tissues swell. This includes clothes, shoes, belts and rings.

Dry burns
1. Move casualty from the source of the burn without harming yourself. (See electrical burns above.)
2. Cover the burn with a clean dressing before calling for help.
3. Continue to reassure the patient and give small sips of water until help arrives.

Fractures

Children's bones are very tough, far more resilient than adults. They often bend rather than snap (the so-called greenstick fracture) and then grow together and heal almost like magic.

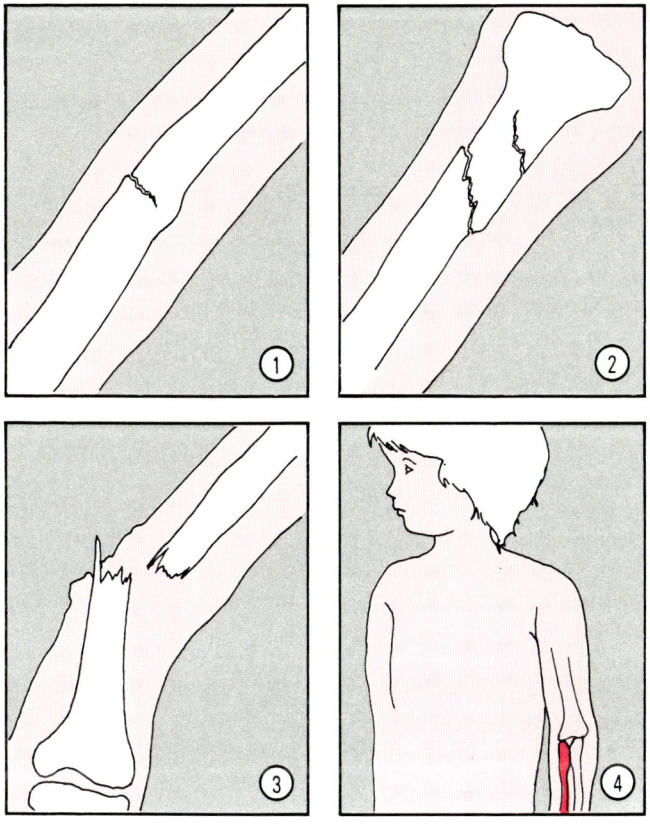

A greenstick fracture (1) and a spiral fracture (2) are both closed fractures. The compound fracture (3) is more serious because the bone breaks through the skin. A pulled elbow (4) is a type of dislocation affecting the radius.

There are about 206 bones in the human body and it is neither possible or necessary for a parent to know all the ways in which they can break. It is often difficult to tell if a bone is broken and the following points are only guidelines. Even a doctor with years of experience may need an X ray to confirm his or her suspicions.

There is one part of the body, however, that needs special mention. Elbow fractures in children can be very serious. If there is any hint of a break, seek medical advice because nerve and blood vessels run close to the bone in this area and can be damaged. If this damage is missed then permanent disability could well result.

A bone may be fractured if:

● There is some deformity. This is easiest to see in broken long bones in the arms and legs if you compare the injured side to the uninjured.
● Your child will not use the limb.
● You can hear the sound of the bone ends grating together.
● There is a lot of pain and swelling in one area.
● You can see the bone sticking through the skin. Living bone is hard and white, exactly as you would imagine. This type of break is called a compound fracture.

What to do
Do not make the injury worse. The edge of a broken bone is very sharp and can easily cut surrounding tissue like blood vessels, nerves and skin. A child may simply return home crying and holding the painful limb in which case take him or her to your doctor or the casualty department. A child that has had an accident and not moved should be left as far as is practical until help arrives. Cover with a blanket and give reassurance. If moving the child is unavoidable, splints and bandages can be used to immobilize and support the injury. Do not touch an open wound. Simply cover with a clean dressing and get help.

If possible gently raise the injured limb to reduce swelling. Put an injured ankle up on a pillow and place a suspected broken wrist carefully in a sling.

Do not give the patient any food or drink. If a bone is broken it is possible the child will need a general anaesthetic at the hospital. If there is food or drink in the stomach the operation may well be delayed until it has emptied because of the danger of inhaling the stomach contents into the lungs while under the anaesthetic.

Dislocation

If the normal arrangement of the bones that make up a joint are distrubed and put out of place, then the joint is said to be dislocated. The joint is usually painful and out of action.

The long limb bones of children have growing points (epiphyses) at the end. A slipping of these areas is more common than the adult type dislocation. This sort of injury is often associated with a fracture and needs urgent medical attention. The longer the tissues remain dislocated, the more difficult the damage is to correct.

A good general working rule is that if a child is still crying inconsolably ten minutes after the injury, then suspect a fracture, dislocation or slipped epiphysis.

Pulled elbow

This is quite a common injury to the elbow and usually occurs in the under-nines. The end of one of the two long bones in the forearm gets pulled out of position. This typically happens when a father pulls the arm either in some horseplay or when swinging the child around by the arm.

Suspect a pulled elbow if after such a pulling accident the child cries and carries the arm limply by the side refusing to use it. The head of the bone, the radius, is easily slipped back without any great fuss or anaesthetic, but it usually needs a doctor to do it.

Poisoning

The first thing to do is to assess the situation. Find out exactly what has been swallowed and ask the child what has happened as soon as you become suspicious, he or she could well lose consciousness later.

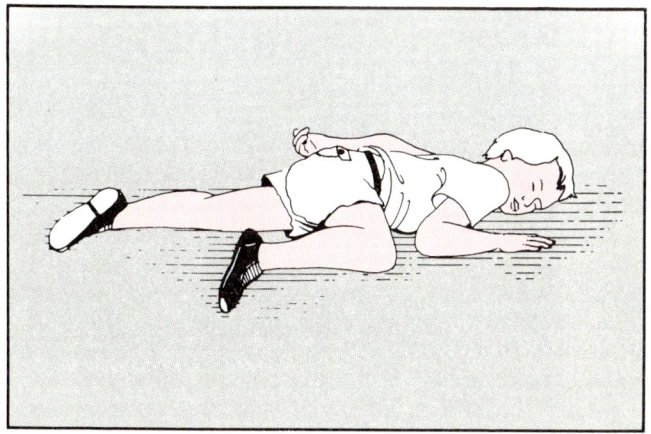

The recovery position is the safest position to lie an unconscious child. The head is to one side so that in the event of vomiting the child does not choke. By placing an arm and a leg at right angles to the body the child will not roll forward onto the face.

Suspect poisoning if:

- There are empty bottles or containers lying around.
- There are burns or blisters around the child's mouth from corrosive chemicals or berries.
- The breath smells of alcohol.
- There are partially ingested berries or seeds in the mouth.

What to do

Remove the child from further harm. Wash any poison out of the mouth, but DO NOT MAKE THE CHILD SICK. Give him or her lots of milk or water and go straight to the hospital. In the time it would take you to make the child vomit, you could have reached the doctor who can give professional advice. Some chemicals do even more damage if they are brought back up again.

If the child is unconscious, place in the recovery position and Dial 999. If you live far away (say more than ten minutes) from the ambulance station and you have a friend with you, it might be worth driving to the hospital yourself. Save all clues to help the doctor decide what and how much has been taken. This means taking any bottles, berries, vomit etc for analysis.

Insect stings and bites

Bites and stings by ants, bees and wasps usually only cause local pain and swelling. It is rare for them to produce the serious problem of an allergic reaction which affects the whole body. You should know what to do if this does happen, however, because it can be life threatening (see below).

Bee stings remain stuck in the skin. If you try to pick it up by the venom sac you will squeeze more down the hollow sting. They are best removed by scraping away from the point of entry with the back of a knife or a fingernail. By brushing the sting out like this, you will not squeeze more poison in if the sac remains attached.

Soothe the pain of the bite or sting with calamine lotion or an antihistamine cream. The alternative is to use dilute vinegar for wasps and ants, and a solution of bicarbonate of soda (one teaspoon dissolved in a glass of water) for bee stings. Apply the cool solution with a compress made from a handkerchief. Rest it lightly on the affected area.

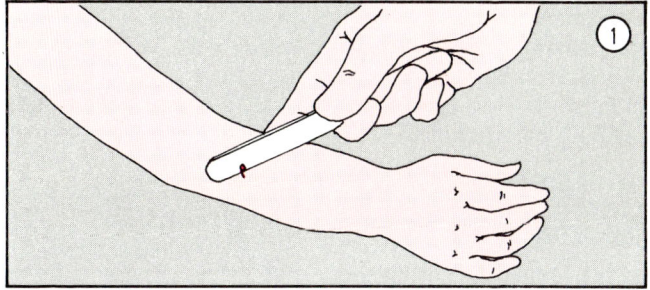

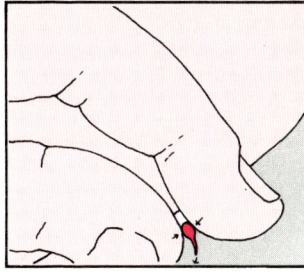

The quicker you remove a bee sting the less poison is pumped under the skin. Scrape it away with the back of a knife or fingernail (1). Do not pinch the sac to remove it because this squeezes more poison into the skin.

Nettle rash (hives)

Stinging nettles stimulate the body to produce the chemical histamine in the skin which produces white, lumpy wheals of various sizes on a reddened skin. The rash is very itchy and may disappear completely after an hour. However, other areas may then come out in the rash and this process can sometimes go on for a few days. Occasionally the child's skin reacts this way to insect bites. The same reaction occurs in response to certain foods and drugs (see Chapter 4 Allergies).

Bites and stings in the mouth and throat should be taken very seriously because swelling could begin to block the airways. Give the child an ice cube or ice cream to suck and get medical advice as fast as possible

With any sting, it is important to keep the child calm because fright and fear can speed up the spread of the venom.

Anaphylactic shock
Very occasionally an ordinary sting can cause a sudden collapse into shock. This is called anaphylaxis and is an form of allergic reaction. It happens minutes after the incident and a collapsed child should be treated for shock (see below).

Treatment
Put calamine lotion onto the wheals and leave it to dry without touching it. This may settle the reaction. The next thing to try is a warm bath with half a cup of baking soda (sodium bicarbonate).

Animal bites

In the United Kingdom there is as yet no reason to worry about rabies (but remember this may not be the case if the bite happens on a holiday abroad) and the majority of children are covered against tetanus from the immunization programme in this country.

It is important, however, to seek help for all but the most minor skin breaks because cats and dogs have many potent bacteria in their mouths and these kinds of wounds very often need antibiotics.

Shock

Shock has many causes. True medical shock is not the same as the shock of something unexpected happening. There is often a misunderstanding about the way the word is used by doctors and parents. True medical shock is a state the body gets into when the blood fails to reach the vital tissues. There are a number of causes.

● **Bleeding**
Blood fails to reach the vital tissues because there is literally not enough to go around.

● **Burns and bad injury**
So much fluid is lost through the burnt skin or injury that the blood circulation (which is part of the body fluid) fails to reach the vital organs.

● **Diarrhoea and vomiting**
If this is severe or goes on for a time without adequate replacement, the body becomes shocked because body fluid is low.

● **Severe allergy**
See anaphylactic shock. Blood pressure falls and so blood fails to reach vital organs.

● **Severe pain or fright**
This is where the layman's term shock comes to be the same as true medical shock. Complicated mechanisms slow down the heart and widen blood vessels so that the blood fails to circulate properly.

Symptoms
The child looks pale, white and sweaty. He or she feels faint, dizzy and sick and the breathing is fast and shallow. The pulse (if you can feel one) is fast and weak. The child may become unconscious.

What to do
Obviously if a child is bleeding heavily, the priority is to deal with the bleeding (see page 137). If this is not the case, lie the child down and raise the legs which brings the blood back to the heart. Move the child as little as possible.

Loosen clothing, especially around the neck and keep the head in a comfortable position but turned to one side which will prevent the inhalation of vomit should the child be sick. Make the child comfortable with a light blanket but do not overheat because this will draw blood to the surface of the skin and away from the vital organs. Do not give anything by mouth in case this causes vomiting.

Hysteria

Some children overreact to unpleasant or stressful situations. It is often worse when there are other people watching. The child may scream, thrash the arms about or fall on the floor. Very often the breathing is unnecessarily fast.

Calm the child down. Be kind and firm without giving excess sympathy. This is best done away from onlookers. Get medical help if it becomes necessary. There is often a need for it anyway; perhaps the child has cut his or her scalp and has been frightened by the blood. Do not slap or forcibly restrain the child.

If breathing is unnecessarily fast, the child may get pins and needles in the hands and feet and around the mouth, although this is more common in adults. The child is breathing out carbon dioxide too fast and should reestablish the equilibrium by breathing in and out slowly from a paper bag held lightly in front of the mouth.

Drowning

If a child is in trouble in water, the first thing you must do is to keep calm and think quickly. Try to reach the child with a stick or a piece of clothing and pull him or her towards you. If you can see the depth of the water, wade in until you can reach with something, and if possible get someone else to hold you. Keep down low so that you do not get pulled over.

What to do

Begin resuscitation as quickly as possible. If necessary this may even need to be in the water. Cold (hypothermia) can complicate the situation so keep the child warm with blankets.

Do not give up trying to resuscitate a child who appears to have died. Children have survived underwater for up to 40 minutes and recovered. They appear to be able to go into a state not unlike hibernation to protect the brain. This is especially so if the water is cold as it very often is. Whatever this process is — and it may be a trick we have inherited from our distant mammalian relatives like the whale which routinely dives under water even though not a fish — do not stop trying to resuscitate the child until you reach hospital.

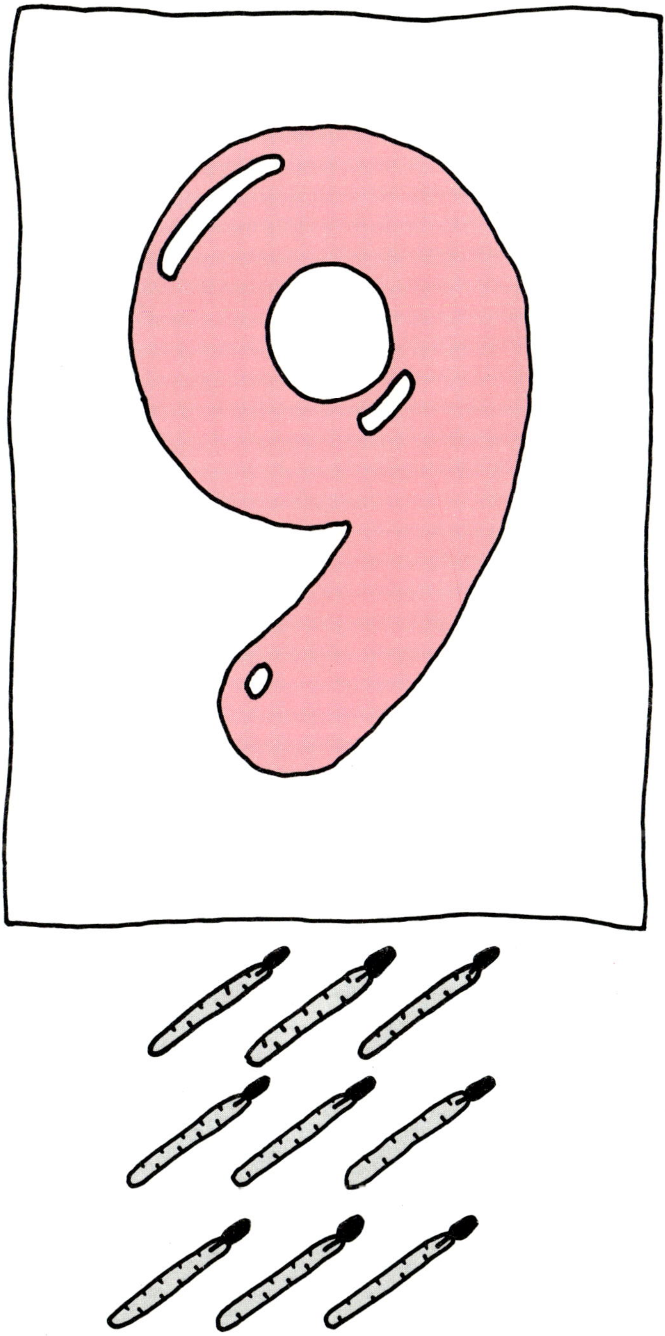

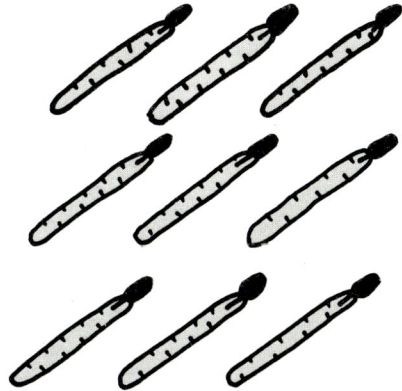

Weight

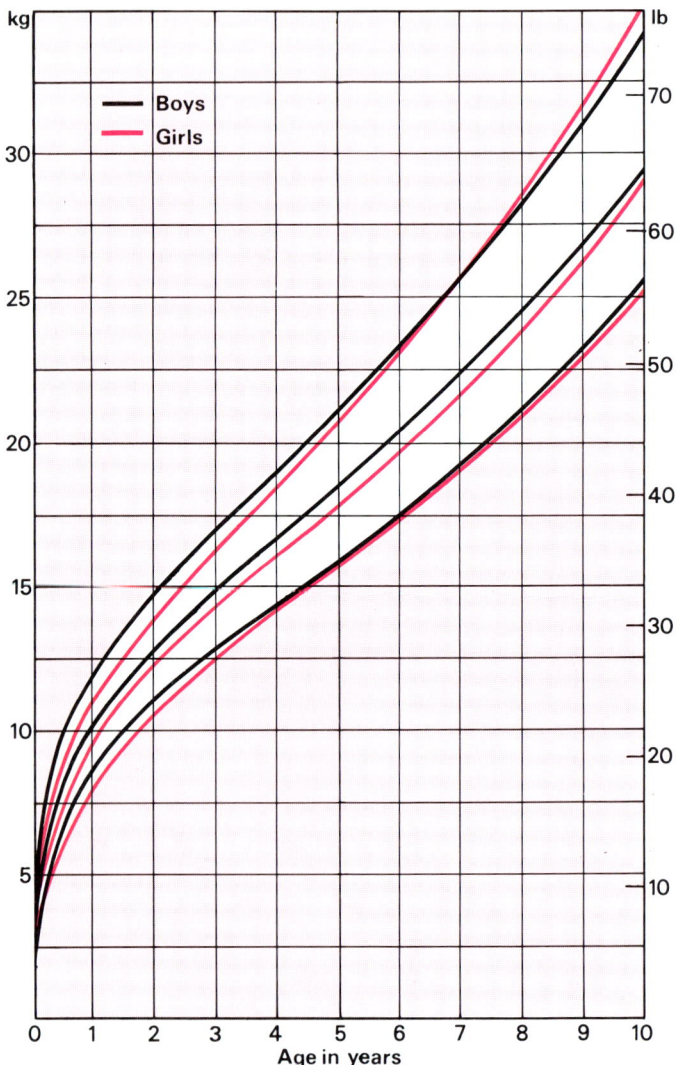

Children's growth is dictated by their genetic make-up and provided they have a balanced diet and good environment during their childhood they will reach their full potential height. Growth can be affected by severe malnutrition but this is hardly ever experienced by children in the Western world. A prolonged period of illness can slow growth, but growth rate speeds up again afterwards to catch up. Growth rate varies for a number of

Height

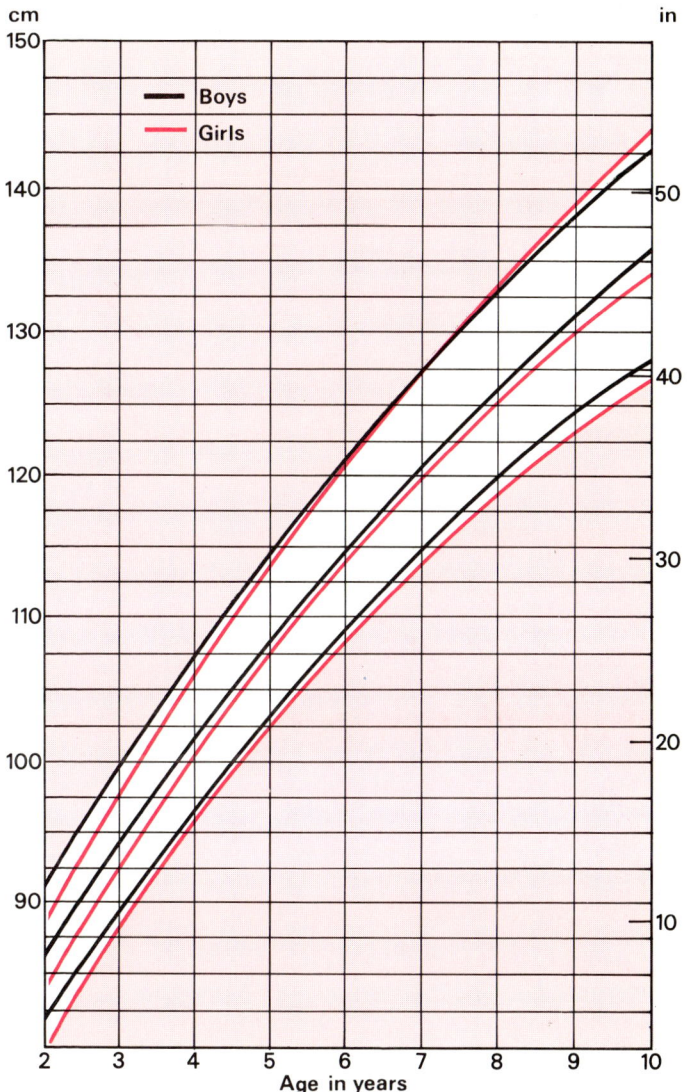

reasons and children should be assessed over a year to see if their growth is normal.

The centre lines of both the weight and the height charts above show the average expected growth rate. The top and bottom lines show the normal ranges above and below this. However, if you have worries about your child's growth, seek advice.

Vaccinations

Disease	Type	Protection
Diphtheria	DPT triple vaccine Injection form	Lifelong
Whooping cough (pertussis)	DPT triple vaccine Injection form	Lifelong
Tetanus	DPT triple vaccine Injection form	Booster required every five years
Polio	Oral vaccine	Boosters required
Measles	MMR triple vaccine Injection form	Not known
Mumps	MMR triple vaccine Injection form	Not known
German measles (rubella)	MMR triple vaccine Injection form	Not known

Useful addresses

National Eczema Society
Tavistock House North
Tavistock Square
London WC1H 9SR

Asthma Society
300 Upper Street
Islington
London N1 2XX

Multiple Births
41 Fortuna Way
Aylesby Park
Grimsby
South Humberside
DN37 9SL

National Association for Gifted Children
1 South Audley Street
London W1Y 5DQ

Play Matters
The National Toy
Libraries Association
68 Churchway
London NW1 1LT

Hyperactive Children's Support Group
71 Whyke Lane
Chichester
West Sussex PO19 2LD

Timing
Three months; six months; twelve months; five years
Three months; six months; twelve months
Three months; six months; twelve months; five years
Three months; six months; twelve months; five years; 16-18 years
Fourteen months
Fourteen months
Fourteen months

Index